HEALTHY HAPPY 100

A Biohacker's Guide to Ageing.

**Heal From Within, Lose Weight
And Look Younger For Longer.**

CURIOUS KIRSTY

ISBN: 9798649020800 (KDP)
ISBN: 978-1-8380842-0-2 (Ingram Spark)

www.curiouskirsty.com

Disclaimer

The following viewpoints in this book are those of Curious Kirsty. These views are based on her personal experiences. She wants to share her journey to fantastic health, in the hope that her readers will benefit.

All attempts have been made to verify the information provided by this publication. The author does not assume any responsibility for errors, omissions, or contrary interpretations of the subject matter herein.

The views expressed are those of the author alone and should not be taken as expert instruction or commands. The reader is responsible for his or her future action. The author does not assume any responsibility or liability on the behalf of the reader of these materials.

This book makes no guarantee of health success.

Contents

GRAB YOUR FREE GIFTS!

There's no point in learning the theory,
if you don't put it into action.

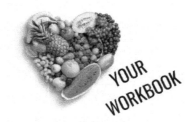

"A Fun Read" · Lise Cartwright

HEALTHY HAPPY 100

A Biohacker's Guide To Ageing

Heal From Within, Lose Weight
And Look Younger For Longer

YOUR WORKBOOK

Curious Kirsty

GRAB YOUR FREE...

HEALTH HACKER 30 DAY CHALLENGE WORKBOOKS

Access them now!

www.curiouskirsty.com/freebies

Follow me on Instagram @curiouskirsty

TAKE THE QUIZ!

How Can You Upgrade Your Health?

Understand where the chinks lie in your health armour.

www.curiouskirsty.com/quiz

DEDICATION

Self doubt is every writer's demon.

Thanks for helping me through the dark times.

PROLOGUE

Shivers shot down my spine as the phone rang. A lump swelled in my throat as waves of dread washed over me as. Trembling, I picked up the phone and took the full force of the blow.

"She's gone".

I knew that my life would never be the same without her. I wept for my loss and for her courageous suffering.

A formidable force of nature, my auntie never complained or showed any sign of weakness as she battled through chemotherapy.

In the grieving process, I found myself asking a hundred questions. In the end, they all came down to the same one, ***why her?***

I regret not being able to share with you the key to living a long and healthy life.

But perhaps I can help somebody like you.

INTRODUCTION

A 2020 article in the Telegraph newspaper read…

"Life expectancy stalls in Britain for first time in 100 years, as dementia toll rises".[1]

If you follow poor advice, you obtain poor results.

Food industries are more concerned with making money than keeping you healthy. When they sponsor research into their own products, the studies are more likely to show favourable results.[2] One tactic is to repeat studies until they achieve the results that meet the objectives of the sponsor. Alternatively, they choose participants who they hope will give them positive results. This corruption has made us mistrust new health advice, as it always seems to contradict the last.

In 1958, American scientist Ancel Keys had a theory; he theorised that saturated fat caused heart disease, and set out to prove it. He started with twenty-two countries, but only included seven in his research.[3] He didn't include countries such as Norway, where people eat a fatty diet but don't suffer much heart disease; or Chile, where they don't eat much fat but have high rates of heart disease. The food industry jumped on board, offering us low-fat options for every imaginable product. They replaced the fat with sugar or artificial sweeteners. While saturated fat—in moderation—is fantastic for your health, sugar and artificial sweeteners are not. The Sugar Research Foundation sponsored Ancel Key's research.[4] Billions of dollars were spent on studies unsuccessfully trying to prove Ancel's theory, and millions of people suffered health consequences.

The Truth Is Out There.

Recent medical breakthroughs have finally revealed how our bodies work. The gut has far greater power than we ever imagined. It affects our mood and immune system, and can even trigger disease. We also know how to prevent diseases like dementia and cancer, or reverse diabetes. The trouble is that hardly anybody knows about these medical advances. The research is tucked away in academic journals, littered with complicated medical terms. Some of these papers are so difficult to read, I wonder if scientists want people to understand their research at all! If health were a jigsaw puzzle, I have pieced it together. I trawled through hundreds of research papers and dozens of health books to offer you clarity on your health. Don't wait another five years for this information to become common knowledge. Give yourself a head start!

You decide upon your health destination.

A decade ago, I studied an undergraduate psychology degree. At that time, we thought that our genetic makeup determined 50% of our health. Now we understand that your genes only account for approximately 25%.[5] The great news is that a healthy lifestyle can override a genetic predisposition. Just because people in your family suffer from cancer and dementia, you won't necessarily get it. You can dodge the bullet by being healthy!

Wouldn't it be wonderful if we could mistreat our bodies, then take a pill to fix the damage? In 2018, Pfizer abandoned the search for an Alzheimer's drug. Brain disease is the result of tiny cuts, which end up as a massive gaping wound. You would need a miracle cure to reconstruct that kind of brain damage. Meanwhile, keeping yourself fit and healthy prevents cancer. You want to equip your body with the power to clear away dead cells, which can become cancerous if they hang around too long.

How I transformed my health without willpower.

The more I learnt about health, the more optimistic I felt about ageing. This optimism turned into enthusiasm, which became a passion. If you are passionate about health, you are naturally motivated to lead a healthy lifestyle. Yet, to be passionate, you must understand how your body works. I have explained complex research in simple terms. I want health science to be accessible to everybody— not just scientists.

I have cracked the health code. The information in this book helped me to heal my aches and pains, lose weight, gain energy, and increase my brain power. I now know just how good my body is supposed to feel. I want to share this knowledge with you. After all, why wouldn't you want to feel fantastic every day?

You can become a biohacker.

A biohacker lives on a different biological timescale. Many are around thirty years younger than their true age. Just like the biohackers, you can turn back your biological clock. You will have more energy and focus. This book doesn't just cover diet and exercise. It gives you a complete overview of health.

If you don't understand food, you can't eat properly. **Understanding Food** answers your burning health questions. What should you eat to live to 100? How much protein do you need? How does your blood sugar work? How do you know if you have good or bad cholesterol? Which fats should you eat? How much alcohol is too much? What are polyphenols and why do you need them? How much salt should you eat? What should you drink and how much?

Discover the food and drink that I use to supercharge my health in **Superfood & Drink;** coffee, tea, ginger, raw honey, organic food, dark chocolate, fermented soy and butter. In **Scary Food & Drink,** you will better understand why you should avoid junk food, artificial sweeteners, energy drinks, industrial meat and milk.

Boost your gut to supercharge your immune system and avoid disease in **Get That Gut Feeling.** A diet can work wonders for one person but not the next. That's because our guts like different food depending on our microbial composition, and our particular food sensitivities. You will find out how to personalise your diet. You will also learn how to test yourself for a food intolerance, and fix your gut lining if it gets damaged. Finally, super-charge your gut with probiotics, prebiotics and resistant starch.

Boost your energy and wellbeing with **supplements.** I will guide you through the research behind the supplements that I take; collagen, whey protein, magnesium, potassium, vitamin D, folic acid, iron, zinc, fish oil, iodine, vitamin C, and copper. Find out why calcium and vitamins E & A do more harm than good.

The best **weight-loss** strategies also prolong your lifespan. Biohackers live by intermittent fasting and a modified Ketogenic diet. Overweight and slim people have different gut bacteria. You will learn how to manipulate your gut bacteria to recreate a slim person's gut. You will also learn how to hack your hunger and why snacking isn't necessarily good for you.

Exercise is a miracle cure for ageing. Find out how to get maximum gains in minimum time. Use your heart rate to get fit quick and get a fantastic workout in 12 minutes. 10,000 steps was fabricated as a marketing ploy to sell pedometers. Learn the real number to aim for, which is backed by research. Understand that standing up lowers your blood sugar, stretching can prevent an injury, and foam rolling improves your posture.

Specialists call Alzheimer's "Type 3 Diabetes". **Avoiding Alzheimer's** is simple if you know how. A particular kind of exercise wards off this brain disease. Learn how to hack your sleep and prevent the herpes virus from spreading into your brain. Nicotine is amazing for an ageing brain. You can ingest it without experiencing the nasty side effects of vaping.

Orgasms are cardio for the brain, and can ward off dementia. sexually active people live longer. That's why I want you to have more frequent and better orgasms. **Healthy, Happy, Horny** will teach you how to combat erectile disfunction and how to locate the G spot. Women are more prone to dementia than men. One reason is that they experience less orgasms. All women can have multiple orgasms; it's inherent in our biology. You are about to boost your libido and learn how to orgasm on demand.

I have tackled the most common conditions that plague our health in **Beat Your Illness**; depression, arthritis, sinusitis, type 2 diabetes, Irritable Bowel Syndrome and allergic diseases. You will discover treatments that even health professionals are not yet aware of.

In this day and age of global virus pandemics, you need a strong immune system. You will boost your immunity and be fighting fit to shake off the next coronavirus in **Dodge A Bullet.** You will also learn how to prevent and sooth lower back pain, combat infertility, and reduce your exposure to blue light. Lastly, find out how giving blood could save your life.

Upgrade yourself by fixing your vision, strengthening your teeth, and harnessing the power of the sun. Meanwhile, you will learn the **healing** techniques that biohackers use; red light therapy, cryotherapy, and grounding. All three decrease inflammation and boost your energy.

Learn how to protect yourself in **Avoiding Toxins.** We are swimming in toxins, but the government is slow to protect us. We can make simple changes to avoid chemicals, endocrine disruptors, and mercury. How you cook your food is as important as what you eat. You will learn which cooking methods to use, which cookware to choose and which fat to employ.

I wrote this book for people who are **frustrated** with conflicting health advice. I want you to be fighting fit and sharp as a knife at 100 years of age. Health science evolves rapidly. This time next year, we will know even more about how to prevent disease. I will routinely update this book. I want to motivate you to stay healthy. When you buy this book, you get **lifetime update** to the latest health news.

How to use this book.

You will better understand where the chinks lie in your health armour when you take the *"How Can You Upgrade Your Health?"* **quiz.** This quiz will give you an idea of which sections will most benefit your health.

At the end of each section, you will find a **Health Hacker 30 Day Challenge** which will kickstart your health transformation. I offer you the workbooks as a **free gift**. You will find them in your first email from me. Focus on one workbook at a time, else you might feel overwhelmed. Every time you start a 30 day challenge, you can stack your new healthy habits upon the previous.

I want you to see the science for yourself, so I have hyperlinked every piece of research cited in this book. I will send you the full **references** via email in case the hyperlink stops working. Otherwise, access them on my website www.curiouskirsty.com, where you can also learn about my journey to fantastic health. Get some health advice from people on the same health journey in the Curious Kirsty support forum.

Your health transformation is about to begin. Get ready to feel better than ever!

UNDERSTANDING FOOD

GET FAT!

Fat doesn't make you fat.

The first myth to bust is that fat is bad for you. Your brain actually needs a regular supply of fat to work at its best. Your brain is 60% fat.[1] So, it makes sense that you need a lot of it in your diet. What's more, essential vitamins A, D, E, and K are only absorbed if you eat fat.

Your brain loves the **saturated** fat in animal products, dark chocolate, and coconut. Sustainable palm oil is another good option. Your brain also loves the **monounsaturated** fat in olive oil, nuts, and avocados.

Some kinds of fat are bad for you. Good fats are blamed for damage caused by sugar and bad fats, such as obesity and fatty liver disease.[2]

Trans fats to be banned in the UK.

Trans fats, labelled as "partially hydrogenated vegetable oils", are often found in processed foods such as margarine, crackers, biscuits, cakes, and microwave popcorn. They are **toxic!** They damage cells, causing strokes and heart attacks.[3] Denmark banned trans fats in 2004 due to the dangers they pose, and by 2016, they saw a great reduction in heart attacks.[4] Food makers manipulate fats to make their products last longer.[5] Trans fats are so bad for you, that they will be banned in the EU from April 2021.[6]

After 2021, don't assume that it's safe to buy junk snacks. It costs too much to make cheap food with quality fat, so these foods are still likely to be terrible for you. If you want to eat cakes and biscuits, make them yourself using butter. If you are lactose intolerant, choose ghee or lard.

Omega-3s are good for your mental health.

There are two kinds of fats; omega-6 and omega-3. Both fats are important, but they do different jobs. When you cut yourself and need to heal, a scab develops and covers the wound. While omega-6 helps to make the scab, omega-3 heals the wound.[7] You need a balance of these two fats to heal, but most people eat far **too many omega-6** fats and not nearly enough omega-3.[8] A healthy fat balance is also important for your mental health. People with psychiatric problems tend to be overloaded with omega-6 fats.[9] The easiest way to consume omega-3 fats is to eat fatty fish, such as mackerel, or grass-fed animal products. The vegetarian options include seaweed, soybeans, walnuts, and flax or chia seeds. The easiest way to cut back on omega-6 fats is to **change the oil** that you use to cook or fry foods. Ditch the vegetable and seed oil and replace it with saturated fat such as butter, ghee, lard or coconut oil.

It can be a **leap of faith** to switch from a low-fat diet to one that includes good fats. I used to eat a low fat diet, and struggled endlessly with my weight. I ditched the bad fats, processed sugar and refined carbohydrates. The weight fell off me. It seemed as though the more good fats I ate, the slimmer I became. Good fats make you feel fuller for longer, so you end up eating less. Also, if your brain is made up of 60% fat, it needs a constant supply to work at its best.

Bottom Line

If you don't eat bad fats or refined sugar, you can eat as much good fat as you like!

PROTEIN

It's true that we need quality protein, but not as much as food companies would like us to believe!

Protein builds muscle. The best sources of protein are meat, eggs, tofu, whey, fermented soy, and nuts. When it comes to protein, you can have too much of a good thing! Too much protein can cause an early death[10] because you are more likely to develop a disease.[11] It's all about **balance**, because too little protein is also bad for you.

Older people need extra protein to stop their muscles from wasting away. Unless you are older, there is **no evidence** that you will benefit from a high-protein diet. Eating too much protein in middle age increases your cancer and diabetes risk.[12] If you are middle aged and worry about the amount of protein there is in your diet, you are already eating enough! Unless you train a lot, you only need two palm-sized portions of protein per day.

Bottom Line

Only older people need extra protein. Food companies want you to believe that you need to eat more protein than is good for you.

SUGAR

Sugar is not necessarily bad for your health.[13]

But… people who eat a lot of sugar and carbohydrates are **more prone** to disease.[14]

We eat far more sugar than we should because we don't understand how much is in our food. And it's in our interest to know, because high blood sugar can cause diabetes and dementia.[15]

Fruit is sugar. People think that the sugar in fruit is better than in a chocolate bar. Truthfully, your blood sugar will spike a similar amount if you drink fruit juice or a hot chocolate. The only thing that will stop your blood sugar from sky-rocketing is the **fibre** in the fruit.

Fruit is much sweeter than it used to be. Because of our sweet taste, fruit has been cross-bred to be extra sweet. So, while fruit has vitamins in it, we should not eat too much. Two portions a day is plenty. Dried fruit spikes blood sugar more than fresh fruit. If you want to be smart, eat your fruit for desert when you blood sugar is already high. The government tells us to eat "five a day" to be healthy. If you want to live until 100, eat **at least** five portions of vegetables and one or two fruit portions a day.

Bread is sugar. Carbohydrates such as rice, bread, pasta, and potatoes turn to sugar in your body. Again, fibre is key. A fibre-heavy sweet potato will spike your blood sugar less than white bread or pasta. If your muscles don't need the energy, the sugar turns into fat and is stored for later use.

Some foods have way more sugar in them than you realise. The biggest culprits are:

low-fat yoghurt,
condiments,
pasta sauces,
readymade soup,
canned fruit,
baked beans,
cereal or protein bars,
smoothies,
flavoured coffee or tea,
vitamin water,
Sports drinks,
granola and cereals.

Tip!

If you eat cereal or toast for breakfast, your blood sugar will spike. Two or three hours later, you will experience a dip, and crave more carbs to lift you out of the dip. Experiment with breakfast options which don't spike your blood sugar so much, such as porridge (oatmeal) or eggs. You can hard-boil eggs for breakfast on the go. Another great option is full-fat natural yoghurt with crushed nuts, 100% cocoa powder and a natural sweetener. — SEE ARTIFICIAL SWEETENERS

Bottom Line

Eating sugar now and again isn't going to kill you. But if you eat too much, it certainly will.

HYDRATION

Hard water is good for you!

Drinking a lot of fluid flushes out toxins from your body and improves your complexion. Women should drink at least **eight** glasses of fluid a day and men should drink **ten.**[16] Symptoms of dehydration are tiredness, feeling unable to concentrate, dizziness, headaches or muscle cramps.[17]

What should I drink?

Have you ever noticed that when you drink loads of coffee or tea you want to go to the toilet? It won't make a difference if you drink one cup, but you will go to the toilet more than normal if you drink a lot.[18] Some people say that coffee and tea don't hydrate you, but that's **not true.**[19]

Hard water comes straight out of the tap (faucet). Hard water is actually better for you than soft water, because it contains more **calcium** and **magnesium.**[20] Drinking hard water saves money and the environment. It's a win-win situation!

Tip!

Adding **bicarbonate of soda** (baking soda) to water hydrates you better than salt water.[21]

Make your own rehydration supplement! Combine 1 tablespoon of sugar, 1/4 teaspoon of salt and 1/4 teaspoon of baking soda in a big glass of water. If you drink it after a heavy night out, you will feel better for it in the morning.

At what temperature should I drink it?

To get your bowel moving in the morning, fill two thirds of a pint glass with tap water, and one third boiling water. Water straight from the tap is better absorbed than hot or cold water, but it doesn't taste very nice. So drink it as you like!

Tips!

Do you have a dehydration problem? Develop a drinking habit! If you drink a glass of water every time you return from the toilet, you will stay hydrated for the rest of your days.

Little and **often** is key. If you drink it all at once it will go straight through you.

Bottom Line

Unless you drink loads of caffeine or alcohol and pee it all out, whatever you drink will hydrate you.

SALT

You need salt in your life.

Too little salt in your diet can be **as bad** for your health as too much. You need salt to keep hydrated, else fluid passes right though you. Eating salt isn't actually bad for you, except if you eat more than 2.5 teaspoons a day.[22]

Why should I eat salt?

Too little salt in your diet makes it more likely that you will develop **diabetes.**[23] Avoiding salt could hurt your **heart**[24] and increase your **cholesterol.**[25]

Processed food contains a lot of salt. If you eat a lot of these foods, you don't have to worry about getting too little salt! Even minimally processed foods contain loads of salt. If you eat a lot of the following foods, you don't need to add salt to your diet:

> ready meals,
> breakfast cereals,
> cheese,
> tinned vegetables,
> readymade soup,
> bread,
> pizza,
> readymade pasta sauces,
> crisps (potato chips),
> bacon,

sausages,

pâté,

cakes and biscuits.

If you don't eat a lot of these food, make sure to season your food with quality salt.

Which salt should I use?

Cheap table salt contains a caking agent that can stop you from absorbing vitamin C.[26] Pink and sea salt contain slightly more minerals than table salt. The big bags of Himalayan pink or sea salt are very affordable. Order online.

Bottom Line

Don't be afraid of salt.

CHOLESTEROL

High levels of good cholesterol is a sign of good health.

Cholesterol is **misunderstood.** Cholesterol is a waxy substance in your blood which you need to build cells and make hormones. The lipid panel test measures three kinds of fat:

- Low-density lipoproteins (LDL). This "bad cholesterol" clogs up your arteries and increases your risk of heart disease. The **lower** the LDL in your bloodstream, the healthier you are.

- High-density lipoproteins (HDL) is "good cholesterol." It transports bad cholesterol from the blood to the liver, where it's excreted. The **higher** the number, the healthier you are.

- Triglycerides are another type of fat in the bloodstream that is stored in fat cells.

Reducing your cholesterol can help you to avoid a stroke or heart attack. People with high cholesterol used to be told to simply reduce their fat intake. But it's not that easy, because you need good (HDL) cholesterol. Good fats increase good cholesterol, and bad fats increase bad cholesterol (LDL). Your doctor may tell you to avoid fats in the first stage of cholesterol reduction. But make sure to re-integrate saturated and monounsaturated fats into your diet at a later stage to increase good cholesterol. The **Mediterranean diet** is perfect. It's full of fatty fish, nuts, olives, fresh produce and extra-virgin olive oil. The Mediterranean diet allows a **little** wheat, red meat and dairy.

How do I know which kind of cholesterol I have?

If you are overweight you likely have bad cholesterol. Unless there is a thyroid issue, people who avoid bad fats don't tend to become overweight. It's hard to get fat on mackerel, dark chocolate, and avocados! If you have high cholesterol and want to reduce it, see PRESCRIPTION MEDICATIONS

Bottom Line

Good fats promote good cholesterol and bad fats promote bad cholesterol.

POLYPHENOLS

Polyphenols make your hair grow!

Polyphenols are antioxidants that **repair** cell damage. You can find them in vegetables, fruits, nuts, dark chocolate, tea, and coffee. Polyphenols **fight disease**, benefit your brain, and can even make your hair grow!

What are antioxidants?

Think of your body as a bike. When the metal is exposed to oxygen over a long period of time, it rusts. Anti-oxidants fight against the oxygen damage. So, if you don't want a rusty body, eat polyphenols!

Polyphenols can prevent **dementia.**[27] If you eat enough of them, they can prevent or help to treat **cancer**.[28] Eating polyphenols helps destroy damaged cells that could otherwise become cancerous,[29] and remove damaged cells at the right time.[30]

Polyphenols increase your metabolism, which makes you burn more calories. They also protect you from heart disease, strokes, and type 2 diabetes.[31] To top it all off, polyphenols even make your hair grow![32]

Eat many **vegetables** such as red onions, spinach, artichokes, asparagus, cherries, strawberries, hazelnuts, and flax seeds. **Grape juice** is packed with polyphenols and proven to help your memory.[33] 100% cocoa powder keeps you focussed,[34] because it has a mild caffeine-like effect.

If you want to increase your polyphenols, you can take a supplement. Anti-ageing experts take polyphenol supplements because they make rats age incredibly well. However, polyphenol supplements deplete iron.[35] If you take **Fisetin,** make sure to get enough iron in your diet from red meat, spinach, or a supplement.

Tip!

Diluted grape juice tastes like Ribena. Kids love it!

Bottom Line

Eat vegetables, fruit, nuts, dark chocolate, coffee, and tea. Take polyphenol supplements if you want to, but watch your iron levels.

ALCOHOL

Drink makes your brain shrink.

Most of us drink too much alcohol. However, **some** alcohol is good for your health.

Why is getting drunk so bad?

The first problem with drinking too much is that it makes you put on **weight.** Apart from eating pure fat, alcohol is the most calorific thing you can put in your mouth. When you drink alcohol, your body stops burning the food you ate and starts burning the alcohol. This makes it more likely that your dinner will turn to fat. The second problem with alcohol is that it makes your **brain shrink**. The more you drink, the more your brain shrinks.[36] In effect, alcohol makes you stupid. Lastly, it damages your stomach lining so that vitamins from food aren't absorbed optimally. For example, alcohol stops you from absorbing folic acid. Women who drink a lot of alcohol are more at risk of developing **breast cancer.** SEE– FOLATE

Resveratrol is a polyphenol famously found in wine. Don't believe the hype. You would have to drink two bottles of red wine to get enough useable resveratrol. You might have fun trying, but it won't do your body any good!

How much is too much?

Everybody is different. If you feel no effects the day after, your body was not overloaded with toxins. Does your mind feel foggy? Do you feel tired? If so, you drank too much. The after effects also depend on what you drink. For me, vodka and gin give me less of a hangover than dark spirits, and white less than red wine. Many people have an intolerance to gluten and don't realise it. So beer makes them feel worse than other drinks. It also depends on **when** you drink. Drinking before bedtime affects your sleep and makes you feel more tired the following day. SEE - SLEEP

People who drink more than one medium glass of wine or beer a day (**14** units per week) are more likely to develop **dementia.**[37]

Why is alcohol good for me?

If you can drink a bit, and **not get drunk**, you could avoid a stroke. Alcohol lowers stress and helps us in social situations. The problems begin when we start to depend on alcohol to relax and enjoy ourselves.

I used to rely on alcohol to have a good time. I had to give up alcohol completely for a few months to get rid of the dependence. Give it a try! You will be a lot less bothered about alcohol when you start drinking again. Although I occasionally drink too much, I have a lot more self-control than I used to.

Bottom Line

Drink a bit, but don't get drunk. If you drink far too much, it is possible that you have forgotten how to have fun and relax without alcohol. Give it up completely for a few months to rid yourself of the dependence.

AGE LIKE THE EXPERTS

If you want to live until 100 years of age, don't stuff your face until you feel sick.

The Okinawan people live on an island near Japan. Until recently, they had the **most centenarians** (aged over 100) than any other civilisation in the world.[38] On average, Okinawan men live to 84 and women 90. They experience **fewer** cases of cancer and dementia than we do in the west, even though there are fewer doctors per person.[39]

What did they eat?

Okinawan people ate, miso soup, seaweed, sweet potatoes, whole grains, and pulses. Pulses include lentils, peas, beans, and chickpeas. They ate a little fish, pork, and tofu for protein, but hardly any dairy products. They also ate many green and yellow vegetables. They drank green and turmeric tea.

The Okinawans have a dinner-time mantra that equates to, "Only eat until you are 80% full"!

Their diet has now changed. They eat **more meat** and **less vegetables**. Nowadays, they have the same life expectancy as the rest of Japan.

Bottom Line

If you want to live to 100 years old, eat and drink green stuff, and don't overeat until you feel uncomfortable.

SUPERFOOD & DRINK

The term — Superfood — is a great marketing ploy. Food companies want you to believe that exotic foods are better for you than the ones in your garden. In reality, weeds and stinging nettles have as many health benefits as those on supermarket shelves.

In this section, I want to give you a taste of the food and drinks that super-charge my diet. Our guts are all unique, and we all have different tastes. A food is only "super" if it works for you. It could be super healthy for one person, but not the next. — SEE GET THAT GUT FEELING

I could write an entire book on superfood and drink alone. If you don't find these ones appealing, research online to find some that you would like to try. Because eating isn't supposed to feel like a chore!

COFFEE

Do you want to live a long and healthy life? Drink coffee!

Coffee is packed with cancer preventing polyphenols. Drinking an extra cup of coffee a day could **lower your risk** of developing diabetes by 11%.[1] It reduces the chance that you will get liver cancer,[2] and Parkinson's Disease.[3] Coffee can **protect you** from heart failure,[4] high blood pressure[5] and bone fractures.[6] It also allows fat cells to release their energy, so it encourages weight loss.[7]

Filter brews are better than instant coffee. Decaffeinated coffees are less good for you.[8] Drink between **three and four** cups a day to get the best health kick.[9] More than five a day is too much.[10]

Beware!

Excessive caffeine during pregnancy can hurt your **baby's liver**[11] and **damage sperm**. SEE– INFERTILITY

Some people feel jittery and wired for hours after drinking coffee. They have a gene adaptation which means that they can't remove it from their bloodstream as quickly as other people.[12] If this is you, **steer clear!**

Tip!

If you drink caffeine as soon as you wake up, your body doesn't release your wake-up hormones. That's why you feel groggy in the morning before your first cup. If you want to feel alert in the morning without caffeine, **wait** half an hour before you take a drink.

Bottom Line

Don't feel guilty about drinking coffee.

ENGLISH CUPPA TEA

Black tea can prevent a stroke!

Black tea is not grown in England, but we call it English tea all the same.

- It reduces **inflammation,** which in turn helps lower high **blood pressure,** protecting your **heart** and reducing risk of a **stroke.**[13]

- It can lower your **blood sugar.**[13]

- It also helps your **brain.** People who drink a lot of green or black tea have brains that are better wired up.[14]

Beware!

Adding milk to a cup of tea can **destroy** the benefits. The proteins in milk (caseins) bind to the polyphenols and stop them from working.[15] If you want to benefit from the polyphenols in tea and coffee, **ditch the milk.**[16] Drink tea with a dairy-free milk, which does not contain caseins.

Tip!

Your sense of **taste changes**. The more you taste something, the more you like it. It took me months to adapt to almond milk. Now, I like it as much as cow's milk. If you hate the taste, Earl Grey tastes good without milk; or drink black tea with a slice of lemon like they do in Spain.

Bottom Line

Tea without cow's milk is amazing for your health.

GREEN TEA

People who drink green tea every day live longer.[17]

- Green tea **protects your cells** from damage.[18]

- It **wakes up** dying cells and removes them from your body.[19]

- It can protect you against diseases such as **arthritis.**[20]

- It's even used as a hand sanitiser to kill bacteria and viruses. If it can do that to your hands, it can also kill off nasty bugs inside you, too![21]

Tip!

Green tea tastes bitter, so add a natural sweetener.

If you don't like green tea, buy green tea **extract** or **matcha** powder. Ask in your local health food shop or order online.

Beware!

It's mildly caffeinated, so don't drink it before bed.

Bottom Line

People who drink green tea tend to live a long time.

ORGANIC FOOD

In 2017, UK farm testing by councils fell by a quarter.[22]

Local journalists went to farms where they found **mistreated** animals that were fed **crap food** like cake and white bread.[23]

The **better** the animal is treated, the **healthier** it is. Grass-fed meat has more CLA than industrial meat. CLA helps to **break down fat**[24] and protects your heart.[25] Organic meat has **less fat** compared to industrial meat. It also has more vitamins A, E and cancer-fighting antioxidants.[26]

Organic eggs are laid by pastured hens. They can roam outside and soak up the sunshine. Organic eggs have **three times** more vitamin D than barn eggs,[27] as well as more vitamin A, E and omega-3 fats.[28]

"Free-Range" might not mean that the hens go outside. The RSPCA says, "Although shoppers believe they're buying higher welfare, most birds sold are **intensively reared** indoors."[29] Look for "Organic" or "RSPA ASSURED" on supermarket labels. Otherwise, go to a local farm shop.

Humans are healthier when they are **relaxed**, and so are animals. The **healthier** the animal, the more **nutritious** it is to eat. To be sure that the animal you are eating led a relaxed life, eat **organic.** On UK organic farms, animals are truly free range. They also enjoy better food and beddings. Remember, whatever the animal eats, you eat.

Ask your local butcher for organic meat, or order online from sustainable farms. Sustainable farms offer great online deals. Of course, it costs more to eat organic. But is £7 really too much to pay for a happy little chicken life? Besides, the more people that eat organic, the cheaper it becomes.

Upgrade Your Seafood

Half of the fish and seafood we eat is industrially farmed.

A fish living in a fish farm feels stressed because it doesn't have space to swim about. If the fish is stressed, the fish meat is less nutritious. The quality of the fish goes down even further if it's really stressed in the time before it's killed.[30] Some fish farmers feed their fish plant and animal products.[31] They might also use chemicals and pesticides. For a healthier dish, eat fish caught at sea.

In the UK we mainly eat tuna, salmon, prawns, and cod. When we overeat species, it threatens their existence. Upgrade your fish to more nutritious options, which also puts less pressure on the natural balance of species.

- Swap tuna for **sardines** or **mackerel.** They contain more vitamins and less mercury.

- **Trout** has all the health benefits of salmon with fewer chemicals and antibiotics.

- Choose **hake, pollock,** or **coley** instead of cod. Coley supports your thyroid, heart, and nervous system.

- **Mussels** are fantastic for your brain, and farming in the UK is sustainable. Plus, they filter out heavy metals from the sea by sticking them to their shells.

Bottom Line

The healthier and happier the animal, the more nutritious it is to eat.

RAW HONEY

Used as medicine since ancient times.

Raw honey comes straight from the beehive. Regular honey is pasteurised, which kills off the yeast. Raw honey contains **thirty types** of polyphenols.[32] Polyphenols prevent cells from being damaged and help to remove dead ones. Diseases caused by inflammation are the **leading** cause of death worldwide.[33] The less inflamed you are, the less likely you are to develop disease.

- Raw honey reduces inflammation and helps you to **heal.**[34] If you put raw honey on a wound, it **heals faster.**[35]

- Put raw honey on **itchy skin** like psoriasis to soothe and heal it.[36] If raw honey can heal wounds on your skin, imagine what it can heal on your insides!

- Raw honey is also good for your **cholesterol.**[37]

- It lowers **blood pressure.**[38]

- It lowers your risk of developing **heart disease.**[39]

- Raw honey is better at curing a **cough** than cough medicine.[40]

- A spoonful in the evening can even help you **sleep.**[50]

Beware!

Don't put it in **hot** drinks or food. You might as well buy the cheap stuff because it won't be raw any more. Add it to full-fat natural yoghurt or oatmeal (porridge).

Tip!

Find raw honey in health shops or order it online. Choose a high-quality brand, because cheaper brands sometimes mix their products with syrup. If you don't like the taste or raw honey, mix it with regular honey, which is still good for you.

Bottom Line

Why eat sugar when you can eat honey?

DARK CHOCOLATE

All you need is love… and chocolate!

Chocolate comes from the seed of the cocoa tree. It contains iron, magnesium, and zinc. Check the ingredients label for **70%** cocoa or more. The higher the percentage of cocoa, the better it is for you.

- Dark chocolate lowers **blood pressure**[51]
- Increases good **cholesterol**[52]
- Reduces **inflammation**[53]
- Helps your **immune system**[54]
- Has a mild caffeine effect that helps you to **focus.**[55]

I knew that dark chocolate would be difficult to find in Taiwan, so I took 20 bars of Montezuma's 100% with me when I went to live there. The first time I tried it, I thought that it was disgusting! **Taste changes**; the more I ate it, the more I liked it. If you only ate dark chocolate, your sense of taste would adapt. When you eat milk chocolate again, you would find it "too sweet".

Beware!

I once made the mistake of eating 100% chocolate right before bedtime. I was awake for ages.

Tip!

Use 100% cocoa powder to make healthy hot chocolate, flavour oats, or add to deserts.

Bottom Line

The more you eat dark chocolate, the more you like it.

FERMENTED SOY

People who eat fermented soy live longer.[56]

Japanese people love fermented soy. They have the longest life expectancy in the world. Fermented soy is a protein, just like beans and peas. Fermentation breaks down the starch, which makes it easier to digest. It also **increases** the nutrients, including iron, magnesium, and potassium. There are three kinds; Miso, Natto, and Douchi.

People who **replace meat** with fermented soy once a week **lower** their bad cholesterol, blood pressure, risk of heart problems, cancer, and diabetes.[57]

It's easy to make.

1) Wash the soybeans and soak them overnight.
2) Drain, then boil or put them in a pressure cooker.
3) Pour the beans into sterilised pots and mix in the Natto (order online).
4) Leave them to ferment.

Tip!

Batch-cook and store it in freezer pots. Watch a YouTube video for the exact recipe.

Bottom Line

Soybeans are good, but fermented soy is amazing.

EAT BUTTER

Butter is great for your health. Hurray!

We were told that butter was bad for us, but we now know that saturated fat is good for us. It was a **terrible idea** to switch to margarine. Margarine contains toxic trans fats which will be banned in April 2021.

Butter is packed with **vitamins** A and K2. It contains **CLA**, which is a special fat that…

- Helps your **immune system**[58]
- Fights **cancer**[59]
- Reduces **inflammation**[60]
- Improves **bone health**[61]

When a cow **grazes outside** in the sunshine, she produces super butter. Grass-fed butter has **5 times** more CLA than grain-fed butter.[62] Grass-fed butter also has more beta carotene (Vitamin A)[63] and **omega 3** fats.[64] If you can't tolerate dairy, switch to **ghee**. Ghee is clarified butter which is virtually free of milk proteins.

Tip!

It's best to keep butter in the fridge, but a nightmare to spread. It's much more spreadable if you shave off slithers with a peeler.

Bottom Line

Look on the label for "Grass-Fed".

GINGER

Ginger can prevent cancer![65]

Ginger also…

- Lowers cholesterol[66]
- Lowers blood sugar[67]
- Is a painkiller[68]
- Improves your memory[69]
- Helps nausea[70]
- Lowers blood pressure[71]
- Has antimicrobial properties, so it can fight a virus[73]
- Relieve symptoms of a cold or sore throat

Make ginger tea, or toss it into stir fries and soups to expand blood vessels and improve **blood circulation.** 1g a day improves the circulation in your hands and feet.[72] It tastes great in a curry or a stir-fry. Sugared ginger is a spicy candy. You can find it in health food shops, or buy the sugar-free version online. If you hate the taste, buy it in supplement form.

Tip!

Find ready peeled and diced ginger in the frozen aisle of your supermarket.

Bottom Line

Ginger is a staple of Chinese medicine, and for good reason!

SCARY-FOOD & DRINK

JUNK FOOD JUNK YOU

Unhealthy diets kill 11 million people per year, which is even more than smoking.[1]

Relatively speaking, we haven't been eating junk food for very long. We have recently found out how bad it is for our mind and body. Besides putting on weight, junk food can affect your **mental health.** It's also **addictive.**

Junk food has a ratio of **2g carbohydrates** to **1g fat**. For example, milk chocolate, macaroni & cheese, buttered popcorn, biscuits, crisps (potato chips), cake, pizza, cheeseburgers, French fries and ice cream.

The only natural food with the same 2 - 1 ratio is breast milk. Your brain lights up when you eat foods with this same ratio, and you **can't stop** gorging.[2] When you eat these foods, your brain releases pleasure hormones, so you get a **rush.**[3] The hippocampus part of the brain stops you from eating too much. It stops working properly when you eat junk food. You **gorge** on it because you don't get the signal telling you to stop. The hippocampus also affects your **memory.** You remember the rush that you got from eating junk food. This makes it less likely that you could resist it when you next see it.

Junk food is the worst kind to eat when you are studying.[4] One of the reasons that children from poor backgrounds tend to get worse grades is because they tend to eat poor quality food.

AGE stands for Advanced Glycation End-Product. Glycation is the damaged sugary browning of your cells. When you fry onions, they get sweeter and turn brown. This same process happens to your cells when you eat junk food or excessive refined sugar. AGE's cause **diabetes, allergies** and **atherosclerosis**, an arterial plaque build-up.[5] Appropriately named, AGE's **age you** prematurely and fast-track you towards **dementia.**[6]

Junk food **damages sperm.** The Western diet includes a lot of processed food and refined carbohydrates such as bread, pasta and cereals. People who eat this way tend to have worse sperm. The more vegetables you eat, the better your sperm quality.[7] SEE - INFERTILITY

Junk food messes with your **eating patterns,** making you want to eat at random times. The effect it has on your brain makes you want to eat **late at night.**[8]

People who eat junk food tend to be more depressed.[9] Junk food contains a lot of salt and hardly any potassium. People with high salt, low potassium levels are more likely to develop **depression.**[10]

Besides junk food, avoid **ultra-processed** food. The more ultra-processed food you eat, the earlier you are likely to die.[11] Examples of ultra-processed food are…sweets (candy), fizzy drinks with sugar or sweeteners, dried ready meals, energy bars, instant noodles, most breakfast cereals, white bread (not freshly baked), 0% fat sweetened yoghurt and chicken nuggets.

There's a **fine line** between junk food and good food. Make home-made **healthier versions**. You can make your own pizza and French fries with quality fat and ingredients. Pizza is great fun for kids to make and homemade French fries are easy with an Actifryer machine.

Tip!

When you eat it often, your body gets used to dealing with the heavy load. If you gave up junk food for a few weeks, you would notice how bad it really makes you feel. Since I became healthy, I feel terrible whenever I eat junk food.

Bottom Line

Put junk food where it belongs, in the bin!

ARTIFICIAL SWEETENERS

Artificial sweeteners can make you diabetic.

Too much sugar is bad for you, but sweeteners are worse! Have you thought about what artificial sweeteners are? Chemicals!

Some people know that artificial sweeteners can interfere with your gut bacteria, but few know about the other health risks that they pose. People who consume a lot of artificial sweeteners are more prone to **cancer.**[12] Artificial sweeteners can make you **intolerant** to sugar.[13] If you become sugar intolerant, you can…

- Put on **weight**
- Develop **diabetes**
- Develop **heart problems**[14]

In my opinion, artificial sweeteners will be banned within the decade. The beverage industry **sponsored** many of the original studies. When invested parties pay for studies, their findings are more likely to be **biased.**[15]

Artificial sweeteners are a toxin. But if you ingest them regularly your body gets used to dealing with them. I cut artificial sweeteners out of my diet. Nowadays, if I drink a coke zero, I get a stomach ache.

Tip!

You can buy natural sweeteners online or in health food shops. Add them to natural yoghurt, oats or hot drinks. The plant extract Stevia is the most well-known, but I prefer Erythritol. It's a natural sugar found in fruit, and the only one not to interfere with your gut's essential bacteria.[16] Plus, it's good for your teeth.[17]

Bottom Line

If you want a coke, drink a coke —not the diet kind with harmful chemicals in it.

ENERGY DRINKS CAN KILL YOU

They give you a boost, but hurt your health.

Energy drinks have worrisome side effects. Researchers are campaigning to ban advertising of high-dose energy boosters until they are proven safe.[18]

- Energy drinks can make your heart beat **irregularly.**

- They can raise your **blood pressure.**[19]

- If you mix it with alcohol, you are more likely to do something stupid to put your life in danger.[20]

- If you drink a lot of energy drinks, they can damage your **kidneys.**[21]

- They can also make you **stressed, sleepy,** and **moody.**[22]

How can they make me stressed?

While 250 mg of caffeine makes you feel awesomely energetic, 500 mg makes you irritable.[23] 500mg is the amount of caffeine that most energy drinks contain.

How can they make me sleepy?

The caffeine megadose in energy drinks can trigger insomnia.[24]

How can they make me moody?

High doses of caffeine can affect your hormones, making you feel anxious and irritable.[25]

Bottom Line

If you want an energy boost, drink coffee! If you want a cold drink, drink an iced coffee.

INDUSTRIAL MEAT

Scientists have found the hidden link between human illness and cheap meat.

Antibiotic use in farming is widespread and common. **Two-thirds** of antibiotics used in the EU are given to animals[26] to **fatten them** and prevent them from **getting sick**. Farmers need to use more antibiotics when they keep animals in cramped living conditions because they are more likely to get sick.

In 2006, the EU **passed a law** that antibiotics should only be used to help an animal when it gets sick. But a **third** of countries still use antibiotics as a preventative measure.[27] When farmers use antibiotics, they are supposed to leave enough time before slaughter to clear them out of the animal's system. But sometimes, they **don't leave enough** time and so the antibiotics end up in humans. The same thing happens with fish; fish farms use antibiotics to prevent infections.

If antibiotics can fatten up a cow, they can **fatten you up,** too! Antibiotics wipe out the gut bacteria that regulate your weight. This makes you put it on.[28] If you take antibiotics, you are more likely to become **obese.**[29]

Superbugs

Because of antibiotic overuse in farming, nasty bacteria can be **transferred** to humans,[30] [31] causing diarrhoea, pneumonia, and urinary tract infections. Fancy a nice bit of **E.coli** with your dinner? That's the **risk** you take when you eat **cheap meat.**

Antibiotic resistance is driven by cheap meat.[32] The more antibiotics used in farming, the more antibiotic-resistant superbugs like MRSA develop. If you ingest MRSA, you could contract a **serious infection.**[33] Because it's resistant to antibiotics, it's difficult to treat. If you want to avoid superbugs, eat meat farmed in your **own country.**[34] If we keep eating cheap meat as much as we do, these superbugs will become much more common. To save humans from superbugs, choose **organic, high-welfare** meat.[35]

Bottom Line

Organic meat and fish is more nutritious and better for world health.

DITCH THE MILK

Milk is good for some, but terrible for most.

Milk contains 18 nutrients, so it should be great for you.

If I wanted to persuade you about the health benefits of milk, I could find hundreds of studies in favour of my view. If I wanted to prove that milk can kill you, I could find hundreds of studies to prove that also.

In February 2020, hundreds of milk studies were reviewed. The study found that...[36]

- Milk is good for you if you have a **bad diet**, because it has many nutrients that you lack.

- It does not prevent bone **fractures.**

- It does not help you to **lose weight.**

- It might give you **cancer.**

- You **don't need** to drink milk to be healthy. You can get calcium — a nutrient that helps build healthy bones—from other foods such as green vegetables, nuts, and tofu. Get your vitamin D from the sun, yoghurt, fatty fish, cheese and eggs.

We used to think that the calcium in milk protected you from potential fractures. Now we know different. Scientists think that the D-galactose in milk causes a breakdown in bone strength which can make you **more prone** to fractures. Women who drink three glasses of milk a day are more likely to sustain bone fractures than those who drink none at all.[37] In fact, the more milk you drink, the more likely you are to sustain a fracture.[38]

Many studies link milk to **cancer.** A recent study reported that one glass of milk a day increases breast cancer risk by **50%.** Three glasses a day increases it to **80%!**[39] Lactose is a sugar in milk. The more lactose you consume, the higher your risk of developing **ovarian cancer.**[40]

Milk messes with your hormones, which can mess up your **skin.**[41] Teenagers with acne tend to drink more milk than teenagers with nice skin.[42] Milk can also worsen eczema and psoriasis.[43] If you want to **heal** your skin, ditch the milk.

65 - 70% of us are sensitive to lactose.[44] In other words, milk is bad for most of us. Lactose intolerance varies from country to country. If your ancestors drank milk, you have less problems digesting it.

The Maori tribe in Kenya live and thrive on cow's milk. Their ancestors have been drinking milk for hundreds of years. They drink **raw milk,** cow's blood, and eat the beef. Raw milk has more nutrients in it than the pasteurised kind.

Why is milk promoted as a health food?

-	Milk used to be better when it was raw, straight from the farm. **Pasteurised** milk does far less for our health.

- Researchers studied dairy **in general**—not milk specifically. Other dairy products, such as yoghurt and cheese, gave the illusion that milk was good for us.

- It depended on **where** the study was carried out. Sweden has a long milking history and low incidence of lactose intolerance. A Swedish milk study would obtain more pro-milk results than one carried out in China, where they only started drinking cow's milk recently.

- The dairy industry **funded** milk studies.[45] Vested interests are more likely to report health benefits, because they sometimes repeat studies until they receive the answers that prove their biases.

It's difficult to come to terms with the fact that milk could be damaging to your health. It has been promoted as a health food all our lives, so we understandably feel cheated.

However...

People who eat no dairy products at all are worse off.[46] Cheese, butter, and yoghurt are much **easier to digest.** Fermentation reduces the lactose, and your gut bacteria love it!

To understand milk, we need to unravel its components. There are three good things about milk, namely:

- It contains **saturated fat** —the fat that your body likes.

- It is rich in **vitamins** and **minerals**.

- It contains **whey.** Whey protein has amazing health benefits! SEE - WHEY PROTEIN

Why is milk so bad though?

We don't know yet exactly what it is that makes milk less healthy.

- If it's the **lactose,** we could drink goat's milk, sheep's milk, or lactose-free milk.

- It could be the effect that milk has on our **hormones.** When pregnant cows are milked, their hormone levels are much higher. So farmers could make sure to only milk cows that are not pregnant.

- It could be because it is **allergenic** and **inflammatory**.

- Or it could be the traces of **antibiotics.**

In reality, it's likely to be a combination of these factors.

Why not try **almond milk?** Or ditch milk entirely. Earl Grey tea tastes better without milk than regular black tea.

OK, but I still don't want to give up milk!

- **Goat's milk** contains less lactose than cow's milk. It's less allergenic and has a different milk protein (A2), which is less inflammatory.[47] Goats milk is richer in iron and magnesium, two essential nutrients which strengthen your bones.[48]

- If you can't be swayed, switch from low-fat to **whole milk**. It has less lactose[49] and more of the good fat that your brain likes. **Organic** milk is richer in vitamins and minerals, and is less likely to contain antibiotics. If you order online, you can get raw, organic milk delivered straight to your door. If you want to avoid hormones, ask the company if they milk pregnant cows.

Bottom Line

Milk is good for the minority and terrible for the majority. In my opinion, it's not a risk worth taking!

If you eat good fats and natural produce, you don't need cow's milk to be healthy.

Access the workbook - Health Hacker 30 Day Challenge -
***Change Your Diet.** Start your journey towards healthy eating today!*

GET THAT GUT FEELING

2500 years ago, Hippocrates said, "Disease begins in the gut".

Now we know that he was right all along.

We used to think of the gut as a digestion machine. In fact, the gut is **integral** to our health, and can affect us in the most incredible ways.

There are trillions of bacteria in your gut. You have a mixture of good and bad strains, depending on what you eat. The **more good** bacteria strains you have, the **less disease** you are likely to experience. Every gut is unique. Your particular bacterial makeup is your "gut microbiome".

Your gut releases chemicals depending on what you eat and drink. If you eat healthy food, your gut releases chemicals that make you **happy** and **fight infection.** If you eat unhealthy food, your gut releases chemicals which make you **sad** and hurt your **immunity.**

The gut plays a **key role** in obesity, diabetes, liver disease, cancer, and dementia.[1]

Fibromyalgia sufferers have different gut bacteria than healthy people.[2] Meanwhile, autistic people tend to have **imbalances** in their gut bacteria.[3] Their **behaviour improves** as their gut health improves.[4] Even the eye disease, **Glaucoma,** starts in the gut.[5]

Your gut controls your immune system. If your gut is not happy, it gets inflamed and can trigger an **auto-immune disease.**[6] This happens when your immune system goes haywire and attacks healthy cells. Examples of autoimmune diseases are diabetes, psoriasis, rheumatoid arthritis, celiac disease, IBS, and multiple sclerosis.[7] Autoimmune diseases like these can be helped via the gut.[8] Symptoms **reduce** when sufferers **change their diet** to fix their gut linings.[9]

Your gut can decide whether you **beat cancer** or not.[10] If you have a variety of good bacteria, you will **respond better** to cancer treatment. If you eat the same, unhealthy food all the time, you have a gut with little diversity. Someone with a poor gut is more likely to develop **colon cancer.**[6] Colon cancer can develop when you consume food that your gut doesn't like over a long period of time, such as junk or ultra-processed food.

How To Have A Bad Gut

Your genes determine some of the bacteria strains,[11] but many things can change your gut microbiome. **Antibiotics** and antibacterial **hand gels** can wipe out bacteria.[12] Doctors prescribe antibiotics too often. Frequent and unnecessary use of antibiotics can cause bad bacteria to grow, which could give you an infection.[13] Overusing antibiotics can **cause** diabetes, obesity, inflammatory bowel disease, asthma, arthritis, and depression.[14] When you use anti-bacterial hand gel before you eat something, the gel is **transferred** on to the food, which ends up in your stomach. Also the Tricoslan is easily absorbed though your hands and can impact your gut.[57]

Tip!

Make your own hand sanitiser. Simply buy the cheapest bottle of vodka you can find. Fill a small spray bottle half-way with vodka, half-way with white vinegar, and a squeeze a lemon into it. Otherwise, order organic hand sanitiser online.

What happens in your **early years** determines your future gut health. Children who are fed a healthy diet, tend to have a better gut microbiome later in life. A poor gut in childhood lays the groundwork for obesity and heart disease.[15] Damage to a baby's gut weakens their immune system, so they are more likely to develop **allergies** and **asthma.**[16] Babies who are given antibiotics suffer **gut damage,**[17] as do those born by caesarean section. After a caesarean, mothers actually smear their vaginal fluid over their new-born baby to boost their bacterial diversity.[18]

What Your Gut Wants

Feed your gut microbes the **right food.** The more **diverse** your gut bacteria, the better. Your gut loves plant foods. If you want a great gut, eat at least **30 plant foods** per week. Eat as much variety as you can. Try new fruits, nuts, seeds, and vegetables. After a couple of weeks, your bacteria will start to change.

Beware!

Your gut **doesn't like** a lot of meat. Experiment with different proteins such as fermented soy, tofu, or peas. Only older people need extra protein. - SEE PROTEIN

We Are Unique

Our guts are unique. We had different diets as children and so did our ancestors. The medications you have taken in the past have also shaped your gut bacteria. Food does **different** things for different people. Two people can eat exactly the same food and have different blood sugar readings. Some people need carbohydrates to feel full;

some need fats. Foods that are healthy for one person are **not necessarily** healthy for another. If a particular food works well with your bacteria, it's healthy.[20] That's why a particular diet works well for some people but for not others.

You might be wasting money on "healthy" foods that do you no good. In the UK, we spend £750 million pounds a year on special foods for our guts. While eating fermented food helps most people, it gives others bloating and headaches.[21] **Pay attention** to what works for you.

The easiest way to know what your gut likes is to get a **gut test.** This tells you what foods to eat and what to avoid. The market leader is US-based **Viome.** You put a sample of your poo in a pot and send it for analysis. If you are diabetic, choose **DayTwo.** They give you recommendations based on blood sugar.

Bottom Line

Eat a variety of plant and fermented foods. If fermented food gives you gas or bloating, don't bother buying it.

INTOLERANCES

The quickest way to get a disease is to fill your body with stuff that it doesn't like.

Symptoms of food intolerances are amazingly **varied.** The most well-known are tiredness after eating, smelly wind, heartburn, a rumbling stomach, or bloating. There are also some crazy ones such as a runny nose or a rash.

Be an intolerance detective. Think back to what you ate to bring on the symptoms. This can be tricky because they can arise hours after eating. You might also be intolerant to a few things.

The most common sensitivities are:

- Lactose
- Gluten
- Wheat
- Egg
- Caffeine
- Histamines - SEE SINUS PROBLEMS
- Food preservatives - SEE SINUS PROBLEMS
- Lectins

Lactose

Lactose is milk sugar, and the most common intolerance. Depending on where you live, up to **70%** of people are sensitive.[22] The most common symptoms are bloating, farting, or cramping after eating dairy. An **elimination diet** is the best way to know for sure. Cut dairy out of your diet and see if your symptoms disappear. Some products, including butter, are naturally low in lactose. You may be able to tolerate some dairy products, but not others.

Beware!

You can give yourself a lactose intolerance by giving up dairy. We are tolerant to lactose when we are born because we drink breast milk. If you didn't eat dairy afterwards, you would lose your tolerance to lactose. I gave up dairy for a few months. When I drank milk again I could feel my heart thumping in my chest; a clear sign of intolerance. It also tasted sour, because taste changes depending on what you put in your mouth. After a while of eating dairy, I built up a tolerance again. Unless you think that you have an intolerance, don't give up dairy on a fad diet. Otherwise, you might develop one.

Lectins

Some people react to a **defensive compound** in vegetables. It's supposed to stop animals (like us) from eating them. Lectins are in **nightshade** vegetables such as tomatoes, bell peppers, eggplant (zucchini) and potatoes. They are also in whole grains and legumes such as chickpeas, beans, peanuts, peas, and lentils. If you want to know if you are sensitive to these foods, eat nothing but nightshades for a day and see how you feel. Pressure cooking and fermenting reduces lectins. For example, soybeans are high in lectins but fermented soybeans are not. You can also reduce the lectins by removing the skin from vegetables.

If you think you might be sensitive to lectins, find out more by typing "Anti-Lectin Diet" into a search engine.

Egg

Avoiding eggs can be tricky. It's in many products, including fresh pasta or baked goods. Also, you might be able to tolerate some eggs and not others. Hard boiled eggs are much harder to digest than soft boiled. If you think you might be sensitive to egg, type into a search engine "foods containing egg" to learn what foods to avoid.

Know For Sure

Go see a **kinesiologist** in your area. They test your muscle reaction to different food and drink. When they put a foodstuff next to your skin that your body doesn't like, your muscles weaken. This might sound to you like complete nonsense, but seeing is believing! I thought that I had a gluten intolerance, but it was actually wheat. Now I can enjoy products that have gluten in them such as oats, barley, and rye bread. Type into a search engine "kinesiologist" and your local area to find a practitioner near you.

You can also get a **food sensitivity test,** but the most accurate kind will set you back around £350.

Beware!

Eating "gluten-free" is **not a cheat** to better health. "Free-from" products can be worse for you than the real thing.[19] If you have a gluten intolerance, eat the pasta made from vegetables instead of the fake kind.

Bottom Line

It can be hard work finding out what you are sensitive to, but it's well worth it in the end.

A LEAKY GUT

You could have the genes for a disease, but never develop it because you never had a leaky gut.

Bacterial imbalances can trigger your immune system, which inflames your gut. This can lead to leaky gut syndrome, where **tiny holes** appear in your gut lining. Small food particles then leak through into your bloodstream.[23] Leaky gut triggers autoimmune diseases, such as type 1 diabetes. A leaky gut occurs just before the disease sets in.[24] Hundreds of unexplained conditions are now thought to be **triggered** by a leaky gut. If you already have an illness, a leaky gut can **worsen** your condition. The brain and the gut are linked, which is why people with depression and anxiety feel worse when they have a leaky gut.[25]

Allergies, ADHD, rheumatoid arthritis, autism, acne, depression, multiple sclerosis, and type 1 diabetes are examples of conditions treated via the gut. Fixing sufferers' guts **improves** their symptoms. That's great news!

Tip!

If you have an unexplained condition, try fixing your gut lining.

What causes a leaky gut?

A leaky gut happens when you consume food or drink that your gut doesn't like. **Stress** is also a factor. You might have noticed that when you are anxious, you can feel it in your stomach.

I had a leaky gut. It caused me to develop a food intolerance. At the time, I was working as a high-school teacher, with a side job at weekends. I was stressed! It all started when I ate a takeaway pizza. The pizza particles leaked into my bloodstream. My immune system thought that it was a foreign invader and attacked it. This caused inflammation and gave me a stomach ache. That means that I was already sensitive to wheat, but never realised it. I had never heard of an adult developing a food intolerance. I kept eating the same food, and got a stomach ache every time.

Fix Your Gut

- **Remove** whatever aggravates it. Go to a kinesiologist to check what foods you are sensitive to or get a food sensitivity test.

- Eat **collagen** - SEE COLLAGEN

- Drink **bone broth** - Watch a YouTube video for the recipe.

- **Stop snacking** - Allow your gut a chance to recover in between meals.

- Increase your **good gut bacteria** - Eat a wide variety of natural and fermented foods.

- Take **aloe vera** supplements - Order online or in a health food shop.

- Eat **raw honey** - SEE RAW HONEY

Bottom Line

You can prevent disease by consuming healthy food and drinks.

PREBIOTICS AND PROBIOTICS

Upgrade your probiotics.

Probiotics are **live microbes** that help your gut bacteria. Probiotics **can't make up** for a bad diet; but they are the icing on the cake to turn a good diet into an **awesome** one. You can find them in fermented foodstuffs such as…

- Full-fat live **natural yoghurt**
- **Kefir** - a super yoghurt, packed with good bacteria
- **Live sauerkraut** - shredded cabbage
- **Kimchi** - a fermented Korean side dish
- **Fermented soy** - SEE FERMENTED SOY
- **Kombucha** - a fermented tea

Tip!

Little and often is key. Drinking a little Kefir every day has more of an impact on your gut bacteria than drinking the whole bottle in one sitting.

Beware!

Probiotics aren't good for everybody.[28] If you start to feel weird, bloated, or gassy after eating probiotic foods, **avoid them.** You might also find that your gut likes some probiotics, but not others.

Don't trust a product just because it says "Good For Your Gut". Check the ingredients label. If there are many ingredients, some of them may not be good for you. Choose the most **natural version** available. Kefir and Kombucha drinks can have copious amounts of sugar in them, which is not good for your gut.

Be sensible. An energy drink is still bad for you, whether it contains kombucha or not.

Tip!

Anything that says **0% sugar** and has a sweet taste is bad for your gut. — SEE ARTIFICIAL SWEETENERS

Probiotic Supplements

You might buy probiotic drinks to help your gut bacteria, but they aren't well absorbed by the gut.[26] Buy **kefir** instead. It does a better job at helping your gut bacteria than those small probiotic drinks.[27]

You might also take probiotic pills to help your gut. The trouble is that different strains work for different people. In the future, you will be able to test your gut and order personalised probiotic strains.[29] Unless you have particular condition to treat, **don't bother** taking probiotic supplements.

However, probiotic supplements **can help** people with eczema, food allergies, diabetes, urinary tract infections,[30] non-alcoholic fatty liver disease,[31] and chronic kidney disease.[32]

For more information about probiotic supplements, see IBS AND ALLERGIC DISEASES

Tip!

Probiotic supplements clear up diarrhoea a day faster than normal.[33]

Prebiotic Fibre

Prebiotics turn back the clock on ageing.

While probiotics are live microbes, prebiotics are the **fertiliser** that the microbes thrive on. When prebiotic fibre is given to mice, their brain and body **get younger.**[34]

- Prebiotic fibre helps you to **absorb minerals** such as iron, magnesium and calcium from food. This can strengthen your bones.[35]

- It keeps your **brain younger** for longer.[36]

- It reduces inflammation and helps your immune system, which can **prevent cancer.**[37]

- Prebiotics change your gut bacteria to help you **lose weight**[38] and keep you feeling fuller for longer.[39]

- Diabetics supplement with prebiotic fibre powder for **blood sugar**[40] control.

Tip!

Taking probiotics to help your gut recover from antibiotics can do more harm than good.[41] However, supplementing with prebiotic fibre powder **does help** your gut bacteria to repopulate.[42]

You can find prebiotic fibre in…

- Cancer preventing **prebiotic vegetables** e.g. leeks, asparagus, artichokes, garlic and onions.[43]

- **Walnuts.**[44]

- **Pearl barley** is a grain like rice. Jazz it up with butter and cheese, or add it to soups and stews.

- **Live sauerkraut** is prebiotic and probiotic, but pasteurisation kills the probiotics. Find the live kind in a health food shop or online.

- Mix **prebiotic fibre powder** with food or drink. Order online or in a health food shop. It will probably be labeled as "Inulin".

Resistant Starch

Resistant starch is resistant to digestion. Because it can't be broken down, your gut bacteria can **feed** on it and multiply. Resistant starch helps **diabetics** to become sensitive to insulin again.[45] It can also lower **cholesterol.**[46]

The best sources of resistant starch are…

- **White rice.** Your blood sugar is lower after eating reheated rice than freshly cooked.[47] To avoid food poisoning, refrigerate or freeze the rice as soon as it cools. The danger arises when you leave it out at room temperature.[48]

- **Plantain flour** or **potato starch.** Add them to food drinks, but don't use them in cooking. The heating process causes it to change so it will no longer be resistant to digestion.

- **Oatmeal** (porridge) is great for your gut. If you leave the oats to soak overnight, it becomes resistant starch. Just don't overcook it the next day.

- **Green bananas** are more resistant to digestion than yellow ones, so they stay in your gut for longer.

Bottom Line

For a gorgeous gut, eat fermented foods, prebiotic fibre, and resistant starch.

If you have a condition that can be helped via the gut, take probiotic supplements.

PRESCRIPTION MEDICATIONS

The effectiveness of your medication depends on your gut microbiome.

Statins lower cholesterol, but they don't work for everybody who takes them. In one study, they only worked for 46% of people. 11% didn't see any reduction in their cholesterol at all.[49] While their genes could have been to blame, it was probably their **gut** microbiome which called the shots.[50] If you have a healthy gut, your medication is **more likely** to work than if you have an unhealthy one.

Your gut affects how well prescription drugs work, and prescription drugs affect how well your gut works. One study found that a third of prescription drugs changed the patient's microbiome.[51] A quarter of prescription drugs killed off at least one strain of their gut bacteria.[52] The **less diverse** your bacteria, the **more unhealthy** your gut.

This can become a downward spiral. If you take a lot of medication, your gut bacteria becomes less diverse. This means that drugs work less well. Meanwhile, you might get side effects, so you take more drugs the tackle them!

Treat The Cause

When you take medication, you are much **less likely** to tackle the underlying issue. People who take medication to lower their blood pressure or cholesterol are less likely to change their diet or do exercise.[53] What's the real problem? In the case of high cholesterol, replace bad fats with good fats, do some exercise, quit smoking and eat foods containing anti-oxidants. — SEE GET FAT, CHOLESTEROL, POLYPHENOLS, EXERCISE

Before you take statins, take **plant sterols.** Plant sterols are the best natural treatment for high cholesterol.[54] That's what they put in margarine to lower cholesterol. Years ago, we were told that margarine was better than butter —terrible advice! Margarine contains **toxic** trans fats, whereas butter contains quality fat. Eat butter and buy plant sterols as a supplement. Find them in a health shop or online. — SEE BUTTER

Take **aloe vera** extract. 500mg twice daily for two months lowers cholesterol and improves **diabetes.**[55] Aloe vera extract also helps your **immune system.** It has even been trialled as a treatment for cancer and **HIV.**[56]

Too much fat around your liver stops you from producing insulin. If you lose the fat, your liver can produce insulin again. Imagine for a moment that diabetics could not inject themselves with insulin. A pre-diabetic would surely lose the fat, else face certain death. Instead, a diabetic lays the groundwork for dementia, as well as countless other health complication. — SEE REVERSING TYPE 2 DIABETES

Plants are nature's medicine. Most drugs come from plants, so **try plants first.** Type your condition into a search engine and "herbal remedy" or "plant medicine". If you are not technology savvy, ask in your local health food shop. If they don't know, ask them to find out for you.

Tip!

Whatever condition you have, exercising, eating more vegetables and reducing your sugar intake is likely to help.

Bottom Line

Tell your doctor that you want to try improving your lifestyle before taking prescription medication.

*Access the workbook - Health Hacker 30 Day Challenge - **Fix Your Gut.** Start your journey towards a gorgeous gut today!*

SUPPLEMENTS

Biohackers take bags of supplements every day.

Most Britons lack key minerals such as potassium, magnesium, and copper. The obsession to be slim has made women in their 20s and 30s particularly **deficient** in iron, calcium, and iodine.[1]

Taking a supplement is a risk **if** you don't understand what it does to your body. Some supplements are dangerous to take if you don't have a deficiency. Calcium, iron, and vitamins A & E can do serious harm if you are not deficient.

One day in the distant future, we will be wearing arm bands with our daily vitamin readings on display. Until then, we will have to work it out for ourselves. I have **researched** each supplement, and decided for myself which ones to take. I will guide you through the research behind the supplements that I take. You can **decide for yourself** if they can help you. If you consider the research, the worst thing that vitamins will do is give you expensive piss.

Don't bother taking **multivitamins.** Studies show that they don't make an impact. Companies tend to put **more cheap** vitamins in it and add only trace amounts of the quality ones. Plus, you couldn't possibly fit the amount of vitamins you need into one pill.

Why should I take supplements?

A person with a terrible diet who takes supplements will **add years** to their life. They will have more energy and become ill less often. Of course, the people who would benefit most from supplements are the least likely to take them.

Even though I have an excellent diet, I still take supplements. I **bulk buy** supplements online —a year's supply of each one at a time. I spend around £300 a year. It's an **investment** in myself. The healthier I feel, the more productive I am. I reap the rewards in increased energy and focus. I feel comfort in the knowledge that I am doing everything in my power to be as healthy as possible.

The supplements listed here are the **basic** ones that offer maximum benefit. If you feel drained of energy and your brain doesn't feel as sharp as it used to, supplements could give you a boost.

Unless you try, you will never know!

Tip!

I sort out my supplements into pill boxes a month at a time. This saves time because I don't have to take one pill out of each packet every day. I leave the box out on my dining room table, to remind me to take them with a meal.

COLLAGEN

Discover the anti-ageing secret.

75% of your skin is made of collagen.[2] Collagen is a protein in your skin, muscles, and connective tissue. Collagen doesn't just keep your skin young; it keeps your **body young,** too.

From the age of 25, your body's collagen production rate decreases. **Sugar, sunbathing,** and **smoking** reduces collagen faster than it should.[3] The less collagen your body produces, the more your skin **sags**, the more your **bones weaken**, and the **thinner** your hair becomes. Women lose collagen faster than men, which is why men age better.

- Collagen lessens **wrinkles** by making the skin more stable and preventing skin cell damage.[4] It also hydrates your skin to make it smoother.[5] For better skin, take 10g a day for 6 weeks.[6]

- Collagen makes your **nails strong.**[7] My nails break whenever I stop taking collagen.

- Collagen **heals wounds** as you produce more healing tissue.[8] It also reduces the associated **inflammation.**[9]

- Collagen fights **cancer!**[10]

- 12g a day helps **arthritis** and **osteoporosis** pain.[11]

- It stops your arteries from becoming **stiff.**[12]

- It helps you **lose weight** and reduces **bad cholesterol.**[13]

Tip!

Take collagen if you are diabetic or pre-diabetic.[14]

Where can I get collagen?

Some foods contain collagen, like gelatine. If you eat jelly (jello) at a children's party, you are eating collagen. Collagen is in animal and fish skin, and **animal bones.** Suck out the bone marrow if you dare, or make grass-fed **bone broth.** Ask for grass-fed cow bones at your local butchers and boil them up. For the recipe, type into YouTube "Grass-fed bone broth". Some supermarkets stock it ready-made, or order online.

Which collagen should I choose?

I buy the powdered version. Marine collagen is made of fish skin. Otherwise, it's made from cow bones. If you buy the type made from animal bones, choose **grass-fed.** Buy it in a health food shop or online. It doesn't matter whether you choose marine or animal collagen; your body can't tell the difference from the collagen that your body produces.[15]

If you are vegetarian, drink **green tea.** It helps you to produce collagen.[16] If you don't like green tea, supplement with green tea extract or matcha powder. You need **vitamin C** to absorb collagen, so eat citrus fruit every day or take a pill for that as well.[17]

Tip!

Get "hydrolysed'", because it's easier to digest.

Beware!

Don't put collagen in **hot** food or drinks. Else it will become useless. Mix it into full-fat yoghurt or a cool liquid.[18]

Bottom Line

Take collagen to look and feel younger.

MAGICAL WHEY PROTEIN

Take whey protein every day —but not too much, else you will die.

Whey protein is what makes milk healthy. Lactose intolerant people can normally tolerate whey because it's easier to digest than milk.[19] If you supplement with whey protein, you can get all the benefits of milk without the **nasty** side effects. - SEE DITCH THE MILK

- 54g of whey protein a day lowers bad **cholesterol** and **blood pressure** by 4%.[20]

- It can be as good as **diabetic drugs** to re-sensitise you to insulin.[21]

- It reduces **inflammation.**[22] Inflammation is terrible for your health and the **root cause** of many diseases.

- It helps people with **stomach issues** such as Inflammatory bowel disease.[23]

- It increases the anti-oxidant glutathione, which prevents **cell damage.**[24]

- It even increases your metabolism, allowing you to burn more calories and **lose weight.**[25]

Tip!

Whey especially helps **older** people.[26] It stops their muscles from wasting away.

I buy **grass-fed**, unflavoured whey protein online. I mix it into my morning oats. It tastes a bit like baby milk.

Beware!

Don't overdose on whey protein to get big muscles. You are hurting yourself. People who eat too much protein in middle age, **die early.**[27]
- SEE PROTEIN

Bottom Line

Want to be healthy and look hot? Take a scoop of whey protein every day.

MAGNESIUM

1 in 5 British women are deficient in magnesium.[28]

Magnesium is in a variety of natural foods such as **green vegetables, fruits,** and **nuts.** There is much less magnesium in the soil than there used to be, so it's harder to get enough from food alone.[29]

- Magnesium helps your **muscles, immune system, heart**, and regulates your **blood sugar**.
- Most magnesium is stored in your **bones**.
- Depressed people tend to lack magnesium.[30] You need magnesium to feel **happy**.
- Take magnesium if you are **sleepy**. It can prevent you from napping.[31]

Taking Magnesium

Supplement with a maximum of 350mg a day. Any more can weaken your bones.[32]

If you have a poor diet, supplement with 350mg every day. If you have a fabulous diet, supplement 350mg every other day or 200mg a day.

Beware!

Poor quality magnesium gives you the runs.

Bottom Line

Eat your greens! And take a little magnesium.

POTASSIUM

Less than 2% of Americans get enough potassium.[33] **A quarter of British women are deficient too.**[34]

You must eat a lot of natural food to get enough potassium. Eight bananas will give you a days worth. You are not a monkey, so drink **coffee** or **tea,** and eat a wide variety of **vegetables.**

People who have high potassium levels **live longer**. Potassium reduces the risk of **heart disease** and **stroke,** while protecting your **bones,** and lowering **blood pressure.** High potassium in your blood means you have a good diet.[35] Meanwhile, high salt and low potassium levels means that you have a terrible diet. If you have a big gap between your salt and potassium levels, you are more likely to die from heart problems. Those with the biggest gap are twice as likely to die of a **heart attack** than those who have more even levels.[36]

High **blood pressure** only affects 1% of people who eat solely natural foods, but **30%** of those who eat the **Western diet**. The Western diet is characterised by refined carbohydrates like cereal, bread and pasta, a lot of meat, dairy and sugary snacks.

People with high blood pressure should lower their salt intake. They should also **supplement** with potassium and magnesium.[37] To reduce blood pressure, white people need 2700mg and black people 4700mg potassium a day.[38]

Beware!

Don't megadose! Too much potassium can cause an **irregular heartbeat.**

Ask your doctor about taking potassium if you have **kidney problems** or if you take **blood pressure** medication.

Don't take potassium if you are pregnant. It increases the **preeclampsia** risk.[39]

Bottom Line

Most people would benefit from taking potassium.

VITAMIN D

People who have good D3 levels are 16% less likely to die from cancer.[40]

Vitamin D comes from the sun. For most of human history, we lived outside. This is one of the reasons that hunter-gatherer tribes are so healthy. With our indoor lifestyle, we are **seriously lacking** vitamin D. You can also find vitamin D in fatty fish, dairy products and eggs.

Vitamin D does wonders…

- People who have enough vitamin D get **less cancer** and **die later.**[41]

- People who have heart disease with high vitamin D levels **live longer.**[42]

- **Diabetics** especially benefit from taking vitamin D.[43]

- It keeps your **gut healthy.** Vitamin D increases your gut microbes, which reduces **body-wide inflammation.**[44]

- Reduced inflammation prevents an **inflamed bowel**[45] or a **lung infection.**[46]

- It helps you to **absorb** calcium, which prevents bone fractures.[47]

How to Get Vitamin D

Stand outside in the sunshine without sunscreen for **15 minutes a day** wearing shorts and a T-shirt.

Take 400 IU of vitamin D3. D3 is **better.** Your body can't tell the difference between D3 and sunshine.

Beware!

Don't megadose on vitamin D. It can hurt your bones.[48]

Tip!

Vitamin D is fat soluble, so take it with a meal containing fat.

Even if you take vitamin D3, you still must **go outside.** The sun offers health benefits that you can't get from a pill. - SEE THE SUN IS YOUR FRIEND

Bottom Line

Take vitamin D3, especially if you don't get sunshine on your skin every day.

FOLATE / FOLIC ACID

Discover why folic acid is so controversial!

When you take folic acid, your body **changes** it into folate. Folate is so important that many countries put it in cereals and bread. You need folate for your **brain, nerves, red blood cells,** and **DNA.** Folate also helps to **remove toxins** such as mercury, lead, and alcohol. Many studies have linked low folate levels to poor health. You need it in your skin to protect you from the **sun.** If you have enough folate, you can prevent **cancer,**[49] **stomach problems,**[50] and a **stroke.**[51]

Folate is **foliage.** The best sources are **green vegetables** such as spinach, broccoli, asparagus, and Brussels sprouts.

The Controversy

Studies show that folic acid reduces cancer risk, but a few say that taking folate can cause cancer.[52] 10 - 15 % white and 25% Hispanic people have a gene mutation where they **can't change** folic acid into folate.[53] If these people take folic acid, their cancer risk **increases.**[54]

When you take folic acid, most of it is converted to folate, but some is **left over.** It can't be broken down and used.[55] It's the left over bits which seem to **cause cancer.** They can cause **circulation problems** or interact with other medications you might be taking.[56]

Taking folate is much **safer** than the synthetic folic acid. Your body can't tell the difference between folate and the natural kind in food.[57] Pregnant women absorb folate better than folic acid.[58]

Should I Take Folate?

One in seven people are folate deficient. **Obese people** and **smokers** are most at risk. **Older people** are more at risk than young people, especially if they live alone.[59] I suppose that people who live alone are less likely to make healthy meals.

Moderate **drinkers** are also at risk. The more alcohol you drink, the less efficiently you absorb folate. Women who drink moderately with good folate levels are **90%** less likely to develop breast cancer than those with low folate levels.[60]

Pre-menopausal women should take folate, especially if they don't eat loads of vegetables.[61]

People who have **stomach problems** are more likely to have a folate deficiency. If you have a problem with your gut, folate might help.[62]

You probably know that pregnant women need folate. Yet, studies show that they should also take it **while trying** for a baby.[63]

How should I take it?

Buy folate, otherwise known as 5-methylTHF or 5-MTHT. There is no evidence that taking too much of folate will hurt you,[64] but it's best not to test the theory! Take as directed.

Beware!

Folate and B12 work together.

If you are vegan, take vitamin B12 and folate together. You do not have to co-supplement with B12 if you eat a lot of animal products.

Bottom Line

Don't take folic acid, take folate.

IRON

One third of pre-menopausal women lack iron.[65]

You need iron to make red blood cells, which transport oxygen around your body. If you are often tired, you might be iron deficient. Iron is not only found in red meat, but also in dark chocolate, soybeans, lentils, beetroot and spinach, of course!

You lose a lot of blood when you are menstruating, which is why so many women are deficient. Female athletes are very likely to be deficient because iron is lost in **sweat**. If a pregnant woman lacks iron, she could have a **premature baby.**[66]

<u>Taking Iron</u>

A pre-menopausal woman who exercises regularly should take 10mg iron a day.[67]

If you have periods, don't exercise, and don't eat red meat, supplement with iron **every other** day.

If you exercise regularly, have periods, and don't eat red meat, supplement daily —but **no more** than 18mg.

If you take iron supplements, you must also take copper and zinc. Copper helps you to absorb iron, and you need a steady zinc-copper balance. I take iron every other day, and a pill that contains copper, zinc, and vitamin c every day.

Tip!

Vitamin C also helps your body to absorb iron.[68]

I check the colour of my poop to see how much iron I have in my body. The darker the colour, the higher your iron levels.

Beware!

Too much iron can kill you. - SEE GIVE BLOOD

If you don't have periods and you eat red meat regularly, **don't supplement** with iron.

Bottom Line

Pre-menopausal women are most at risk of iron deficiency. Take an iron supplement unless you eat loads of red meat, especially if you exercise regularly.

ZINC

Two thirds of the global population are mildly to moderately zinc deficient.[69]

Zinc is present in many foods but only in small quantities. If two-thirds of people are deficient in zinc, a third have a good diet full of quality protein, vegetables, nuts, seeds, and grains.

- Zinc helps children to **grow.**[70]
- You need zinc for your **immune system** and to attack **cancer** cells.[71]
- It helps your **memory.**[72]
- It shortens the length of **a cold.**[73]
- Take it if you have skin problems like **acne.**[74]
- It stops your **eyes** degenerating.[75]
- Zinc helps **depression.**[76]
- It helps **diabetes.**[77]
- Take it if you get **diarrhoea.**[78]

Take no more than **40mg** per day. If you take zinc, take **copper** too. Excess zinc depletes copper.

Beware!

Zinc can interact with arthritis medications and antibiotics. Consult your doctor if you are taking these medications.

Bottom Line

You lack zinc unless you have a varied diet full of vegetables, nuts, grains and seeds.

FISH OIL

Fish oil prevents heart attacks.[79]

Fish oil can also prevent **dementia.**[80] Omega-3 fats DHA and EPA reduce **inflammation** in your brain.[81] A reduction in brain inflammation also reduces your **stroke** risk.

While DHA is good for your **memory**, EPA treats **depression.**

- Fish oil also improves **sperm** quality. - SEE INFERTILITY

Eat fatty fish such as **mackerel, sardines,** and **herring.** You might be surprised to know that tinned sardines improve with age. Don't take notice of the expiration date!

Tip!

Some fish oil is pretty useless at helping your heart.[82] Make sure that at least **500mg** is made up of EPA and DHA.

Ask in a health food shop or search online.

Beware!

Check that it's **mercury free.**

Bottom Line

Unless you eat loads of fatty fish, take quality fish oil.

IODINE

Brainy people take iodine.

Iodine is in seaweed, seafood, dairy, prunes, and eggs.

- Take iodine for peak **brain power.**[83] It can prevent brain **damage** by helping braincells to renew themselves.

- It helps your **immune system.**[84]

- It helps your thyroid to produce **hormones.** After the Chernobyl nuclear disaster, people took iodine supplements to protect their thyroid from nuclear damage.

Take iodine if you are **pregnant**[85] or do a lot of **exercise.** You lose iodine in sweat.[86]

Tip!

Buy roasted seaweed—a popular snack in Asian countries —to snack on. You can also add it to your dishes.

Beware!

Don't overdose on iodine in a quest to become a genius; your thyroid might take a hit.[87]

If you have thyroid problems, ask your doctor before taking iodine.

How to Take Iodine

I take 200 micrograms (ug) **kelp** —which is a seaweed supplement. Otherwise, you can buy iodised salt. Order online or ask in a health food shop.

Bottom Line

Take iodine for a sharp brain. Pregnant women and fit people benefit the most.

ANTI-OXIDANTS

Have you ever wondered why hangovers become worse with age? You produce fewer antioxidants as you age, so recovery takes longer. Antioxidants keep your **cells healthy** by protecting them from damage.

VITAMIN C

Shortens a cold by one day.

1g a day (1000mg) Vitamin C shortens the duration of a cold and reduces flu-like symptoms.[88]

Vitamin C helps your **metabolism, immunity, hormones,** and **blood flow.**

You need plenty of vitamin C to make **collagen.** Collagen strengthens your hair, skin, bones, and nails. If you don't have enough vitamin C, your body doesn't have enough to make collagen. It uses it to prevent cell damage instead.

Find vitamin C in **citrus fruits** and **vegetables** such as broccoli and peppers.

Your body can't store vitamin C, so we must get a continual supply. I take zinc + copper + vitamin C in one tablet.

Tip!

If you get a cold, ramp up the dose to at least 1000mg.

Bottom Line

Better to have too much than too little! Any excess will pass in your urine.

COPPER

Copper kills cancer cells and makes cancer treatment work better.[89]

Soil has been depleted of copper so it's difficult to get enough from food. To get enough, you would need to eat seafood, vegetables, nuts, whole grains, and dark chocolate.

If you often feel **tired** or if you have high **blood pressure**, you could be copper deficient. You need copper to produce **collagen** and to absorb iron.

- Copper boosts your **immune system.**

- Your **brain** also needs copper. It helps people with Alzheimer's and Parkinson's disease.[90]

I take copper + zinc + vitamin C in one tablet. I take iron with it because I don't eat a lot of red meat, I have periods, and do regular exercise.

Tip!

If you take turmeric for cancer prevention, take copper with it. Copper helps you to absorb the curcumin, which is the active ingredient in turmeric.[91]

Bottom Line

You lack copper unless you have a fantastically varied, healthy diet.

BEWARE OF CALCIUM

Calcium can give you dementia and cancer.

The most well-known source of calcium is dairy products. Calcium is also in fish like **sardines** or other fish that is eaten with the bones. You can also find it in green **vegetables, tofu,** and **fermented soy.**

People take calcium for healthy bones, but recent studies show that it does **more harm** than good. If you are not deficient in calcium, taking it increases your **cancer risk.**[92] It also increases your risk of developing **dementia** by four times![93]

Instead of calcium, take…

- **Magnesium,** which prevents bone fractures.[94]
- **D3** helps you to absorb calcium from food.
- **K2** helps your bones.[95] Take D3 and K2 at the same time.
- Grass-fed **collagen.**

Bottom Line

Unless you are trying to correct a deficiency, do not take calcium. Once corrected, **stop** taking it.

BEWARE OF VITAMIN E & A

Don't take these vitamins!

Vitamin A and E are antioxidants, which protect your cells from damage. Theoretically, they should make you live longer. However, they stop your **blood clotting.** They also interfere with your **natural defences.**

Beta-carotene is another form of vitamin A. Beta-carotene, vitamin E, and high doses of vitamin A make you **die earlier** than you should.[96] Even taking vitamin E for a **short time** can be damaging.[97]

Find them in natural sources...

- **Vitamin A** is in organ meats, fish oil, eggs, and vegetables.
- **Vitamin E** is in nuts, seeds, quality oils, dark green vegetables, avocados, and kiwis.

Tip!

Vitamins A and E are both **fat soluble.** The danger of eating a low-fat diet is that you can't absorb them from food.

Bottom Line

Don't take these vitamins! Eat good fats, nuts, and green vegetables.

Give your health a boost with a month of supplements.
Access the workbook - Health Hacker 30 Day Challenge - SUPPLEMENTS

WEIGHT-LOSS

Half of British people have recently tried to lose weight, and two-thirds diet most of the time.[1]

INTERMITTENT FASTING

The diet that even slim people do.

Intermittent fasting (IF) is restricted eating within a **specific window.** It's not just people who want to lose weight who do intermittent fasting. Many people do it because it gives them **more energy** and helps them to **think clearly.**

When animals eat in a specific window, they are **less disease** prone and **live longer.**[2]

Here's why…

- IF reduces **body-wide inflammation,**[3] which could otherwise trigger disease.

- Your gut microbes like to **rest** in between meals.[4] Your gut controls your immune system. If you have a happy gut, you have a healthy immune system.

- When your body is not busy breaking down food, it can **clear** out dead cells, and **repair** damaged neurones.[5]

IF Methods

The most popular intermittent fasting method is the 16:8. You only consume calories during **8 hours** of the day. You can choose the window yourself, for example 10am - 6pm or 11am - 7pm.

During the 16-hour fast, you drink black **coffee** or **tea.** If you don't like black coffee, dilute it with hot water and sweeten it with a natural sweetener like erythritol. Earl grey tea tastes good without milk. Herbal tea is also fine. It only takes 15 calories for your body to snap out of fasting mode. Before you ask… yes, alcohol counts as calories!

You might only need a slight adjustment in your routine to reap major health benefits. **Build up slowly.** Push your breakfast back and your dinner forward every day until you are within the window. I clean my teeth after dinner, so I'm not tempted to eat anything.

If you can't manage an 8-hour window, a **10-hour** eating window still helps weight loss, lowers blood pressure, and cholesterol.[6] If you are diabetic, eating two big meals a day is **better** for your blood sugar levels than eating six small meals.[7] Diabetics should make their eating window **earlier,** as skipping breakfast is bad news for your blood sugar.[8] For example, 9am - 5pm would be a good option.

The first thing you will notice is the whole-body **detox.** Your body had the time and energy to clear out the waste which might have been stuck in your bowel for years. It happened to me on the fourth day of intermittent fasting. You will feel lighter than ever!

You can also do the **5:2** diet, which is also good for diabetics.[9] Eat a normal, healthy diet for 5 days and only **600 calories** per day for 2 days **back-to-back.**

The French have a saying "L'appétit vent en mangeant", which means, "The more you eat, the hungrier you are". The reverse is also true. The less you eat, the less hungry you are.

Although I was obsessed by IF when I started, it soon became part of my normal routine. It improved my relationship with food. I learnt that I didn't have to eat every time I was hungry. Beforehand, I would fret about being hungry, and take snacks with me wherever I went! Now I appreciate being hungry, because I know that I will enjoy my meal more. I also found ways to subdue my hunger. — SEE SNACKING BUSTED

I stopped doing the 16:8 diet because I wanted my hunger back. Eating is far less enjoyable when you're not hungry.

Beware!

If you start to feel unwell, **eat something.**

We are all different. Some people get on really well with IF, and some people don't. For example, you might have an irritable bowel that hates being hungry. Fasting should make you feel better, not worse.

Don't do intermittent fasting if you have an unhealthy relationship with food or if you are underweight.

Don't try it if you are pregnant. Babies need a regular nutrition supply.

Bottom Line

Eating a late breakfast and an early dinner is good for your waistline and your health.

THE ONE AND ONLY CRASH DIET

It makes you live longer.

Some people who try the **Ketogenic** diet have bounds of energy and focus. Their aches and pains even disappear.

Ketogenic or "Keto" diets are extremely low in carbohydrates and sugar. Only **1%** of your food intake comes from carbohydrates. It cuts out anything which turns into sugar in your body. You can't eat **wheat, rice, potatoes, nuts, sugary fruits** (e.g. bananas) and **sugary vegetables** e.g. carrots, peas, and sweetcorn. Of course, you must also cut out **refined sugar.**

This is **not** the Atkins diet. Replacing carbohydrates with protein makes you lose weight in the short term, but eating loads of meat is bad for your gut. If a food isn't good for your gut, then it's not good for you. - SEE GET THAT GUT FEELING

If you have ever been on a high fat - low carb diet, you know that carbohydrates keep you hungry. Your blood sugar spikes and dips a lot, so you need to eat more carbs to **lift** yourself out of the dip. You **won't** be as hungry on a Keto diet as you normally would be. A low carbohydrate diet also **reduces cravings.**[10]

Ketosis happens when your body switches from burning sugar to **burning fat.** The liver makes sugar from scratch,[11] which your brain uses for energy.[12] Your brain really **likes** this fuel.[13] People with brain issues reduce their symptoms when they eat this way. It helps people with Autism, Alzheimer's and Parkinson's disease to have a **better**

quality of life.[14] The Ketogenic diet can also stop children from having epileptic fits and reduce the frequency of adult seizures.[15] It works it's magic through the gut microbiome.[16]

Beware!

People who do Keto for a long time **die early**[17] because it stops you from responding to insulin.[18] When you don't eat sugar or carbs, you don't need to produce a lot of insulin and your body stops being sensitive to it. Not producing enough insulin is **as bad** as producing too much. Both can cause type 2 diabetes, among other health problems. If you keep eating 1% carbs, you can't burn off all the fat, which can lead to **diabetes**.[19]

Keto reduces body-wide inflammation. That's a good thing, because inflammation triggers disease. To get the health benefits of Keto without the deathly side effects, do Keto **six days** a week, and eat **quality carbs** on the seventh day. Examples of quality carbohydrates are rice, oatmeal (porridge), quinoa, and potatoes. Biohackers insist that eating this way will make them live a **very** long time.

Keto Tips!

- Keep your gut bacteria happy with **prebiotic fibre powder.** High-protein, high-prebiotic fibre snacks keep you fuller for longer, so you snack less.[20] Take some almond milk or full fat natural yoghurt. Mix in a spoonful of prebiotic fibre powder, a spoon of whey protein, and a spoon of collagen powder. Mix or shake! - SEE PREBIOTICS AND PROBIOTICS, COLLAGEN, WHEY PROTEIN

- **MCT oil** helps ketosis. It's a concentrated version of coconut oil. For best results, buy c8 or c10 oil.[21] MCT has a laxative effect, so take it easy!

- If you want to check that you are in ketosis, you can pee on a Keto stick and check the colour. Order online.

Don't do Keto if…

You are breastfeeding or pregnant. Babies need carbs.

Consult your doctor if you are on antidepressants, blood pressure or diabetes medication.

To learn how to become Keto, type into a search engine "The Ketogenic Diet"

Bottom Line

Your body needs fewer carbohydrates than you think it does.

HACK YOUR GUT

If you are overweight, your gut bacteria could be to blame.[22]

Fat and thin people have different strains of gut bacteria.[23] Some people think that the best way to lose weight is to eat less food. Actually, the best way to lose weight is to **change your gut** to a slim person's gut. To encourage the right bacteria strains, you must eat the right food and drink the right beverages.

To get the gut of a slim person, eat and drink **polyphenols.** Polyphenols are in vegetables, fruits, coffee, tea, and dark chocolate. The more polyphenols you eat, the slimmer you become. Just don't eat too much dark chocolate, it contains sugar after all. - SEE POLYPHENOLS

You can also take the polyphenol supplement **Fisetin,** which is a polyphenol in fruits such as strawberries and grapes. Fisetin makes rats age incredibly well. It is currently being trialled on humans. If it makes humans age as well as rats, we will all be taking Fisetin every day!

Rhubarb extract also encourages slim bacteria,[25] as does reducing your **alcohol intake.** - SEE ALCOHOL

Encourage good bacteria to grow by taking **prebiotic** fibre powder and eating **resistant starch.** You can also eat **probiotic** and prebiotic food. SEE - GET THAT GUT FEELING

Tip!

Avoid artificial sweeteners. Sugar is better for you than these chemicals. SEE - ARTIFICIAL SWEETENERS

Bottom Line

Slim, healthy people eat a lot of vegetables and don't drink a lot of alcohol.

SNACKING BUSTED

Being hungry is good for you.

Snacking myths are peddled by food companies who want you to eat more than you should.

Your gut microbes like to **rest** between food. If you stop snacking, your gut will be happier. If your gut is happy, you are healthy. - SEE GET THAT GUT FEELING

Snacking myth 1 - *Snacking makes you burn calories.*

False! Your metabolism does not speed up when you snack.[26]

Snacking myth 2 - *Snacking keeps your blood sugar steady.*[27]

False! If you are hungry for your dinner, your blood sugar stays lower after you have eaten it.[28]

Snacking myth 3 - *If you don't snack, you will eat more at mealtimes.*

False! You will likely eat a little less, but not a lot. By snacking, you will eat more calories than if you just ate your meals.[29]

Beware!

Avoid snacking late at night. It makes your digestion worse the next day.[30]

Instead of snacking, try these hunger busting tips…

- Sometimes, you are actually just **thirsty.** Drinking 1.5 L of water a day helps weight loss because it suppresses your appetite.[31] When you feel a hunger pang, drink a glass of water. If you are still hungry 20 minutes later, eat something.

- Hunger rears its ugly head when you are **bored.** Distract yourself by changing activity. If you are still hungry 20 minutes later, eat something.

- Drink **coffee** or **Mate.** If you have been to Argentina or Uruguay, you know about Mate. Mate is a green tea made from leaves like the coca leaf, otherwise used to make cocaine. Just like cocaine, Mate subdues hunger. It also contains antioxidants and keeps you focussed. Order online, and watch a YouTube video of how to prepare it. Add a natural sweetener to taste.

- Smelling **peppermint** reduces appetite. Drink peppermint tea, clean your teeth, chew some xylitol gum, or sniff essential oil.[32] SEE- CHEW GUM

- **Exercise** reduces cravings for sugary snacks. Even taking a brisk walk can do the trick.[33]

Bottom Line

Don't snack because you think you should.

*Access the workbook - Health Hacker 30 Day Challenge - **WEIGHT-LOSS** Start your weight-loss journey today!*

EXERCISE

Seventy-year olds who have been jogging for many years are around 30 years younger physically than their biological age.[34]

Want to stay young? **Get fit!**

The three pillars of fitness:

Aerobic exercise: This is where you get **out of breath.** Anything that gets your heart pumping is aerobic exercise. That could be jogging, swimming, cycling, using a skipping rope, or doing star jumps. If you have not done exercise for a long time, walking fast could be enough.

Muscle strengthening: The easiest way to strengthen muscles is to use weight machines at the gym. You could also do sit-ups and push-ups at home.

Stretching: Exercise tightens your body. You are more likely to get injured if you don't stretch. Most gyms run stretching classes, or join a beginner's yoga class. Don't worry boys; men do yoga these days! Plus, you might get a nice view…

The Miracle Cure For Ageing

We have known for a long time that exercise does simple things like lowering blood pressure. But it can do the most amazing things for your mind and body. Exercise is a **miracle cure** for the ageing body and a **must do** for anybody who wants to **turn back** their biological clock.

- Aerobic exercise switches on **healthy genes** and switches off bad ones.[35]

- It makes you **smarter.** The hippocampus is the memory centre of your brain. Aerobic exercise protects it from shrinking and can even make it **grow.** This protects you from a foggy memory and **dementia.**[36]

- Exercise boosts your **immune system** which protects you from viruses.[37]

- It boosts **testosterone** for both sexes. Hormones are great for your sex life. - SEE HEALTHY, HAPPY, HORNY

Glutathione is an antioxidant which **protects cells** from damage. When you exercise, your body produces more glutathione.[38] This **protects you** from toxins, dementia, lung damage, and heart attacks.[39]

- Exercise helps **asthma** sufferers. Asthma worsens if you don't have enough glutathione in your lungs.[40]

- Glutathione **reduces with age.** Older people can keep their glutathione levels topped up with exercise.[41]

- Glutathione detoxifies your **liver.** Exercise does wonders for people who drink a lot of alcohol.[42]

Muscle Strengthening

High blood sugar **damages cells.** Exercise prevents the damage by burning up excess sugar in your bloodstream. In this way, regular exercise **prevents diabetes.**[43] Muscle strength training is especially good for diabetics - SEE REVERSING TYPE 2 DIABETES

When it comes to muscle strengthening, it **doesn't matter** if you spread the workout over the week, or do it all in one day. You can lift a weight 60 times in one day and get the same results as if you lift it 30 times on two separate days.[44]

The fastest way to get strong is to use a weight that is **80%** of the amount you could lift at one time.[45] Find the weight that is so heavy that you can only lift it once, then take roughly 20% of the weight off. You should only be able to lift it between **8 and 12** times.

If your goal is to become strong, one set is enough. Hop from machine to machine in **13** minutes and be nearly as strong as someone who spends an hour lifting weights. The key is to work **incredibly hard** for those 13 minutes; if you're not suppressing a grunt, you're not working hard enough! If your goal is to get big muscles, do a **few sets** on each machine.[46] The more sets you do, the **bigger** your muscles will grow.[47]

Inexperienced older people build muscle as well as experts of the same age.[48] Just **once a week** is enough to obtain major health benefits. Join a gym and ask the staff how to use the weight machines.

Exercise Tips

- Listening to **fast music** makes you go faster![49]

- Get a good night's **sleep**. Sleep reduces post-exercise inflammation and boosts growth hormones.[50]

- Muscle is built in **recovery.** There is no point doing weight training every day.

- **Stretching** is as important as exercising. Stretch in between gym days and your body will thank you for it. If you won't stretch, go **swimming**. Swimming lengthens your muscles and makes you more flexible. Front crawl and backstroke are the best for flexibility.

- **Build up slowly.** You get bad muscle ache when you start to train. **Don't worry!** Your body will get used to it and you won't feel it as much. I like to have a bit of muscle ache the day after. It makes me feel like I worked really hard.

Debilitating Conditions

People with debilitating conditions used to be told not to exercise. Not only does exercise **reduce pain**, but it makes sufferers more mobile and **less depressed.** When people with Parkinson's Disease participate in exercise, their **symptoms improve** and they can lead a more normal life.[51] A **combination** of exercises works best for people who have depression and fibromyalgia.[52] That's aerobic, muscle strengthening, and stretching.

Exercise is great for your **spine.** It regenerates nerves and strengthens back muscles.[53] It rehabilitates a spinal cord injury.[54] If you have a **back problem,** book an appointment with a physiotherapist and ask which exercises would help you.

My Experience

I exercise because it makes me feel fantastic. If I work out in the morning, I feel relaxed and energised for the entire day. My brain feels sharper, and I can concentrate for longer. When you start working out, you will likely feel worn out. **Don't give up!** You will soon start to feel fabulous.

I wouldn't say that I enjoy weight training, but I love the feeling I get afterwards. Besides, it only takes 20 minutes. You don't have to spend hours in the gym to get strong! I enjoy running and swimming. There's something therapeutic about concentrating on a routine activity. I experience clarity of thought, and get fabulous ideas whilst working out.

I find that my body changes most when I change activity. If you do the same exercise, your body adapts to it. When you change the kind of exercise you are doing, your body has to work extra hard.

Tip!

If you find the monotony of running dull, join a team sport like netball or grass hockey. The comradeship will motivate you, and you will make some new fit friends.

I am writing this book in Covid-19 lockdown. When businesses resume, many workers will benefit from more flexible working hours. Why not ask for an extra 30 minutes for lunch? You can make it up at the end of the day. Then you can pop to the gym and come back feeling refreshed and energised.

Bottom Line

If you want to age backwards, combine the three pillars of fitness. Do at least one session of each a week.

STAND UP FOR YOURSELF

It's not sitting at work that will kill you, it's sitting at home.

If you sit on the couch for **4 hours** a day, you have **50%** more chance of developing heart disease than someone who sits for 2 hours. You are also more likely to suffer an **early death.**[55]

If an inactive person walks for half an hour, they cut their risk of an early death by **17%**. If that same person walks briskly so that they are out of breath, they cut their risk by **35%**.[56]

Watching screens makes you **depressed.** The more time you spend watching television or staring at a phone or computer screen, the more depressed you are likely to be.[57] Any more than two hours watching programs per day is bad for your mental health.

Standing up instead of sitting down after a meal lowers your **blood sugar** by 11%. - SEE REVERSING TYPE 2 DIABETES

Instead of sitting on the couch...

- Learn to **juggle!** Juggling is wonderful for your brain. Whenever I want to learn a new skill, I watch YouTube videos. Buy 6 balls so that you don't have to bend down to pick them up every time you drop one. You can also let your couch catch the balls.

- Learn to poi. If you don't know what poi is, take a look of the videos on my website or Instagram. www.curiouskirsty.com #curiouskirsty

- Do some **housework.** You would be surprised at how many calories you can burn running the vacuum cleaner around.

- Do some **stretching.** Leave the TV on in the background if you like.

- **Stand up** and call a friend.

- Start a **garden.**

- Stand at a high table and do a **jigsaw puzzle.**

- Do some **batch cooking** for your freezer.

Bottom Line

Any more than two hours a day sitting watching a screen is bad for your brain and body.

HIIT

10 minutes of exhaustive exercise gets you fitter than 50 minutes jogging at a steady pace.[58]

High Intensity Interval Training (HIIT) is **short bursts** of intense exercise. Between the bursts, you take a short rest or do gentle exercise. There are countless ways to do HIIT. You can mix muscle strength training and aerobic exercise. In a 20-minute session, you could do star jumps for 2 minutes, rest for 30 seconds, do some push-ups, and repeat. To get the best results, don't rest for more than **one minute.**[59]

HIIT could be as quick as a **4-minute** Tabata training session. Tabata is eight intense sets of 20 seconds with 10 seconds rest in between. The more sets or 4 minutes you do, the fitter you become. Type Tabata into YouTube and follow some workout videos.

HIIT Benefits

- HIIT boosts **testosterone** and **Human Growth Hormone** (HGH).[60] It protects you from fractures, builds muscle, and gives you energy. You start losing HGH at **middle age.**[61]

- **Telomeres** are the caps at the end of each **DNA** strand. They protect DNA, as plastic tips at the end of shoelaces stop the string fraying. As you age, your telomeres wear away and your DNA becomes damaged. Exercise keeps your telomeres long and strong, which makes it **less likely** that you develop disease. Older people with long telomeres are physically **9 years** younger than their biological age.[62]

- HIIT reduces the hunger hormone leptin. You are **less hungry** afterwards.[63]

- Compared to other exercises, you burn **more fat**, and in less time.[64]

HIIT For Type 2 Diabetes

When you eat sugar, your body releases insulin to get it out of your system. If you eat too much sugar, your body releases too much insulin. Your organs become desensitised and don't react in the same way to insulin as they used to. HIIT helps your organs to **re-sensitise** to insulin. Your organs are more sensitive to insulin for **two days** after training.[65] Tabata routines are especially good for diabetics.[66]

Bottom Line

HIIT is the most efficient way to get fit.

USE YOUR HEART RATE

A tool to get fit quickly.

Your **maximum heart rate** is the maximum times that your heart can beat in one minute. It naturally declines as you age.[67] People used to work out their maximum heart rate as the number 220 minus their age, but that formula **doesn't work.** There is a new formula, which is more accurate, but not exact.

Maximum heart rate = 208 - (0.7 x age in years)

To get an accurate reading, download a heart rate monitor application on your phone. **Cardiio** is free— note the double i. Take off the cover and place your finger over the camera at the back for a reading. Most peoples' resting heart rate is between 60 - 80 BPM. If you exercise a lot, your heart gets stronger and you need less beats per minute to pump blood around your body. The fitter you are, the lower your resting BPM.

To measure your maximum heart rate, run on a treadmill. Every three minutes, make it go faster and run on a steeper incline until you can't run any more. Measure your heart rate on your phone. That's your maximum. If you are unfit, walk on a treadmill instead.

When you work out, you want to be at **85%** of your maximum heart rate or more. The closer to your maximum, the fitter you become.[68] People used to say that trying to reach your maximum heart rate was dangerous, but that theory is now disregarded. Just build up slowly if you have an underlying health condition.

HIIT + Heart Rate

If your maximum heart rate is 170, you want to know 85% of that number. Type on a calculator, 170 x 85% = **144.5**

You can have a fantastic workout in **12 minutes** on an exercise bike. Warm up for a couple of minutes, then alternate between cycling hard and peddling slower every minute. In the fast parts, your heart rate should be above **144.5 bpm.** You can measure this on your phone in one of the slower minutes. Always cycle slowly for a couple of minutes afterwards to cool down.

If you are working below **50%** of your maximum heart rate, you are **not getting fit.** If you are working below **60%**, you are **not burning fat.**[69] We used to think that working at a low heart rate was best to lose weight. That's not true! The higher your heart rate, the more calories you burn.[70]

Your maximum heart rate declines with age, so re-measure it every year.

Bottom Line

Using your maximum heart rate will get you fit quick.

STRETCHING

Stretch to avoid a hip replacement.

Exercise tightens your muscles, so you need to loosen them up to prevent injury. Some gyms run stretching classes, or you could join a beginner's yoga class.

To **progress fast,** stretch for 20 seconds, 3 times. In total, you stretch each muscle for 60 seconds.[71] Between stretches, stretch the opposite muscle. If you only hold each muscle once, stretch it for **30 seconds.** The muscle stretches most between 15 and 30 seconds.[72] You make more progress by stretching the muscle twice.

Before you stretch, do a 5-minute **warm up**. Anything will do! Do some star jumps, jog on the spot, walk up and down the stairs a few times, or circle your arms.

You will be more flexible on one side than the other. We tend to be stiffer on our dominant side. It also depends on which way you crossed your legs as a child. Spend longer on the stiff side to even yourself up.

Tip!

You can learn everything on the internet. Type "stretch" into YouTube and the body part to stretch, for example arms, back, hips, legs, neck. Copy the video.

Bottom Line

Stretch at least twice a week.

FOAM ROLLING

Foam rolling is good as a warm up, but it doesn't help your muscles to recover.[73]

A foam roller looks like a big rolling pin made of foam.

People roll over it to massage their muscles and recover from exercise. However, studies report that they are **wasting their time.** However, it can **prime** your muscles for stretching.[74] Your muscles stretch more after massaging them on a roller.

I wish I knew this before. I had a knee problem and spent years rolling out my quadriceps. It didn't help, and now I know why! Nowadays, I only use it for posture. To find out how, type into YouTube "Foam rolling posture upper back".

Tip!

Buy a cheap foam roller online.

Beware!

Unless you are a specialist, don't roll out your lower back. You might cause yourself an injury.

Bottom Line

Foam rolling warms up your muscles for stretching and helps to correct your posture.

10,000 STEPS IS TOO MUCH

Find out the real magic number.

You don't need to walk 10,000 steps to be healthy. This number was fabricated by a Japanese company in order to sell pedometers.

If you walk briskly, **8000 steps** a day is enough to keep fit.[75] Elderly people who walk between 8000 and 10,000 steps have **fewer** heart problems.[76]

Older women who walk **4400 steps** a day stay alive longer than those who take 2700 steps.

Older women who walk **7500** steps or more live the longest. Walking any more than 7,500 steps makes no difference to their lifespan.

Bottom Line

8000 steps a day is the real magic number. You get much fitter if you walk quickly.

7500 steps is the magic number for older people.

*Access the workbook - Health Hacker 30 Day Challenge – **Exercise***
Start your fitness journey today!

AVOIDING ALZHEIMERS

You don't have to lose your marbles. Keep them in play for longer!

There will **never** be a cure for dementia. Brain diseases such as Alzheimer's are a result of **tiny cuts,** which end up as a massive gaping wound. The only thing you can do is limit the cuts so that you never develop dementia. The more nerve cells and neurones are damaged and lost, the quicker you descend into dementia. Some people's brains deteriorate quickly, and some slowly. A healthy brain can become an Alzheimer's brain in just **five years.**[1] The good news is that even people who have the genes for dementia can **dodge the bullet** with a healthy lifestyle.[2]

To look after your brain, you must look after your **body.** People with high **blood pressure** are more likely to develop dementia.[3] If you can't pump blood around your body, **less oxygen** reaches your brain. **Obese** people[4] and those with type 2 **diabetes** are also much more likely to get it.[5]

Increasing **forgetfulness** or "senior moments" is the first sign of dementia. This means that you need to sort yourself out… fast!

TYPE 3 DIABETES

Sugar is the leading cause of dementia.

If your blood-sugar levels spike too high, your liver can't produce enough insulin to remove it from your bloodstream. High blood sugar, means **high brain sugar**, which can damage your braincells. Your brain power also slows down. People who eat too much sugar have **similar** brain damage to people with dementia.[6] The **higher** your blood-sugar, the **faster** your brain will decline.[7] That's why specialists call Alzheimer's **Type 3 Diabetes.** In the long term, the **less** your blood sugar fluctuates, the **smarter** you are.[8]

People with Alzheimer's, Parkinson's Disease and Epilepsy have difficulty using sugar as their brain's energy source.[9] When they stop eating refined carbohydrates such as bread, cereal and pasta, their symptoms reduce.[10] Their brain's prefer ketones, which the liver makes from scratch. To produce ketones, you have to massively reduce your carbohydrate intake. - SEE THE ONE AND ONLY CRASH DIET

To keep your brain sharp, eat the **Mediterranean diet**.[11] In Spain, they eat lots of good fats such as fish, avocados, olives, olive oil, and butter. They eat many vegetables and some fruits. Typically, they eat little dairy, red meat, wheat and drink a little wine. **Antioxidants** protect cells from sugar damage, so they can protect you from dementia too. Antioxidants are in vegetables, fruit, nuts, coffee, tea, and dark chocolate. - SEE POLYPHENOLS

In all the food groups, fats raise blood sugar the least.[12] For a healthy brain, eat **good fats** such as eggs, cheese, nuts, coconut, and seeds. Brainy dessert options are fruit, dark chocolate and full fat, natural yoghurt. - SEE GET FAT

Tip!

People with Alzheimer's disease tend to have low selenium levels.[13] Eat **Brazil nuts**.

Bottom Line

Dodge dementia by eating fresh, natural food. Meanwhile, limit refined carbohydrates and sugar. - SEE SUGAR

GET OUT OF BREATH

Aerobic exercise helps your brain to process sugar for a week![14]

Aerobic exercise is the kind where you get **out of breath.** - SEE EXERCISE

The **fitter** you are, the better your **memory**, and the **less likely** you are to develop dementia.[15] Unfortunately, getting fit won't help you if you already have it.[16] So, get fit **now.**

When you exercise, your brain produces chemicals that stop brain damage.[17] Exercise after brain injury helps to **repair** the damage[18] and **protects neurones.**[19] People who have had a stroke or spinal cord injury especially benefit from aerobic exercise.

The fitter you are, the bigger your brain,[20] and the more **intelligent** you are. The less active you are, the more your **brain shrinks** and the more likely you are to develop dementia.[21] Both yoga and aerobic exercise make you smarter, but **only** aerobic exercise prevents dementia. Aerobic exercise **flushes away** plaque that destroys neurones. This prevents the hippocampus from shrinking, and your memory from deteriorating.[22]

Ideally, train 4 times a week for 40 minutes at a heart rate of **85 - 95%** of your maximum. - SEE USE YOUR HEART RATE

If that sounds like too much, aim for **1 hour 30 minutes** aerobic exercise a week. Every little counts! Even one session a week helps your brain.

Exercising **throughout** your life protects you from dementia. Unfit 18-year olds are more likely to develop early-onset dementia than fit people.[23] An unfit older person who improves their fitness extends their life expectancy by three years and prevents dementia by two.[24] If you start doing aerobic exercise now you will probably **never** get it!

Tip!

Orgasms are **cardio for the brain**. They bring a rush of blood to your brain, and vital nutrients along with it. - SEE HEALTHY, HAPPY, HORNY

Bottom Line

The more aerobic exercise you do, the less likely you are to develop dementia.

DRUG ABUSE IS BRAIN ABUSE

If you abuse your body, you abuse your brain.

You might not think of tobacco and alcohol as drugs, but they **wreck** your brain.

Stop smoking! Smokers are laying the groundwork for dementia. However, there is some good news. If you quit, your brain can **fully repair** the damage and your increased dementia risk disappears.[25]

To ensure that your brain is fighting fit, drink no more than **14 units** of alcohol a week.[26] That's a pint of 4% beer or medium glass of wine a day. No.... You can't save them up and get slaughtered on a Saturday night!

Protect your brain with these supplements...

- **Moringa** leaf extract restores healthy neurotransmitters.[27] Buy this South-American power plant in powder form online. Add it to your food or drink. It tastes a bit like asparagus.

- Taking **curcumin** every day improves memory and mood in older people with memory loss.[28] Curcumin is the active ingredient in turmeric. However, it's unlikely to be absorbed properly.[29] Take it with a meal containing **fat, copper,** and **bromelain** (a pineapple extract).

Tip!

Don't combine it with black pepper extract. It can **hurt your liver.**[30]

Bottom Line

Alcohol and tobacco lay the groundwork for dementia. Healthy food and aerobic exercise **prevent dementia** and make you more **intelligent.**[31]

HERPES

Herpes medication prevents dementia.

Two-thirds of people under 50 have the herpes simplex virus. If you ever had a cold sore, you have the herpes virus. Most people show **no symptoms** and never know they have it. If your grandma kissed you with a cold sore as a child, your immune system was strong enough to fight off the symptoms. If someone with a cold sore kisses you as an adult, you get cold sores. If someone with a cold sore kisses you down below, you get genital herpes.

Once you catch it, you can never rid yourself of it. Even though I don't get cold sores anymore, I know I still have the herpes simplex virus. The trouble is that it can spread around your body and into your brain. People with dementia are **more likely** to have the herpes virus in their brain.[32] In fact, if you have the virus, you are more than **twice** as likely to develop dementia.[33]

Acyclovir and other antivirals treat genital herpes. If you take Acyclovir, your risk of dementia goes down.[34] In one study, people who took a single long and high dose of acyclovir were **10 times** less likely to develop dementia.[35] Antiviral drugs don't cure herpes infections, but they stop it from **multiplying** and contain the spread. This reduces internal inflammation which prevents brain damage. Besides dementia, the herpes virus can also trigger schizophrenia, epilepsy and fibromyalgia.[36] Fibromyalgia sufferers,[37] epileptics[38] and schizophrenics are more likely to develop dementia.[39]

Anti-aging experts say that viruses are doing far more damage to our brains than we realise. They take an anti-viral like Acyclovir every year to prevent the damage.[40]

Beware!

Anti-virals can interfere with medications. If you are on medication, consult your doctor. Be especially cautious if you have kidney problems.

If you don't want to take Acyclovir, take the natural version. **Moringa** leaf extract restores healthy neurotransmitters and can prevent the herpes virus from entering the brain.[41] Order Moringa powder online and add it to food and drink.

Bottom Line

Take a course of acyclovir every year or add Moringa to your diet.

SLEEP

The best health tonic money can buy, and all it will cost you is time.

The more quality sleep you have, the **less nerve damage** you sustain, and the less chance you have of developing Alzheimer's.[42] When you don't sleep well, you damage nerve cells.[43] People who suffer from Alzheimer's disease have a lot of nerve cell damage.

Sleep helps your brain **wash away toxins.**[44] As your sleep quality deteriorates, so does your ability to clear out these harmful toxins.[45] The more toxins in your brain, the more chance you have of developing Alzheimer's disease.

You don't sleep to save energy; you sleep to **heal.** The amount of energy you use while you sleep only reduces by **a quarter.**[46]

- Sleep boosts growth **hormones** and reduces stress hormones.[47]

- Sleep boosts your **immune system**.[48]

- People who sleep poorly are more likely to become **obese.**[49] When you sleep badly, you feel terrible. When you feel terrible, you want to eat junk to make yourself feel better.

- Sleep makes new **memories**.[50] It allows the brain to process what happened that day.

- Quality sleep makes you emotionally stable and happy.[51]

Sleep Myths

MYTH 1 - *Older people need less sleep.*

Older people need **as much** sleep as young people. But getting quality sleep becomes more difficult **after 60** years old.[52] As you get older, your brain releases more stress hormones. As you might expect, stress makes it harder to fall asleep![53] Older people also produce less of a hormone called "melatonin", which means that you are less sleepy at bedtime.[54] Older people should take extra care to get quality sleep. If they sleep badly over a long period of time, they have a **44%** higher risk of heart disease.[55]

MYTH 2 - *You can catch up on sleep.*

Once you have a bad night sleep, the nerve **damage is done.** You can't repair it the next night.[56] The only way to reverse the damage is to take a **long nap** the same day.[57]

MYTH 3 - *Alcohol helps you sleep.*

Alcohol gives that impression, because you fall asleep quicker; but the quality is **worse.** You get less deep restorative sleep. Alcohol won't affect your sleep if you finish your drink **4 hours** before bedtime. If you get tipsy at lunchtime, you still get quality sleep.[58]

How much should we sleep?

People who sleep between **7 - 8** hours do better on tests.[59]

People who sleep 9 or more hours a night have a 23% higher risk of **stroke**[60] and a 14% increased risk of **death.**[61] People who sleep for 10 hours have a **30%** increased risk.

6 hours a night should be a bare minimum.

Napping

Healthy people seldom nap. Frequent napping is either a sign of poor-quality sleep or an unhealthy lifestyle.

If you sleep more than six hours and still need a nap, you are more likely to have a **stroke** or **heart attack.**[62] If you take long naps (90 minutes) you have a **25%** higher risk of stroke.[63]

Tips!

Set an alarm for **30 minutes.** If you sleep for longer, you go into a deep sleep, and feel groggy for the rest of the day.

Take **magnesium**. It can prevent you from napping so that you sleep better at night. - SEE MAGNESIUM

Raw honey in the evening can improve the quality of your sleep. - SEE RAW HONEY

Circadian Rhythm

This is your **natural sleep rhythm**. I tend to sleep from 11pm - 7am. Some people are night owls; some get up early. We used to think that staying up late was bad us, but now we know different. It **doesn't matter** when you sleep, if you get **quality** sleep. Still, staying awake all night isn't good for you. People who work night shifts are more likely to develop cancer.[64]

Your internal sleep clock **shifts** as you age. Teenagers have a different circadian rhythm, which is why they **sleep later** in the morning. Teenagers need to sleep until 8am to get enough deep sleep. Schools in the US that change their school hours to later in the day achieve better academic results.[65]

Whatever time you sleep, make sure to have a **regular bedtime.** Older people who don't have a regular bedtime are more likely to develop heart disease.[66]

Tip!

Light receptors in the skin help to regulate your internal clock. Get some sunlight on your skin in the **morning** to reset your sleep clock.[67]

Blue Light

Electricity is a relatively new invention in human history. When we see light, our bodies think that it's day time. The more bright light you see in the evening, the less sleepy you become.[68] If you have a dimmer switch, lower the light intensity. **Dim** the brightness on your phone and computer screens. Fluorescent light is the **worst kind,** and red bulbs are best. Why not put some red bulbs in your bedroom? They might create a sexy atmosphere…

Tip!

Buy some yellow tinted, "blue blocking" glasses to wear in the evenings. You don't realise how much your eyes are straining until you start wearing them. Order online.

Healthy People Sleep Better

Health and sleep influence each other. Quality sleep makes you healthy, and being **healthy** promotes quality sleep. If you eat well[69] and do regular exercise,[70] you will enjoy better sleep than unhealthy people. Vegetables, dairy products, fish, and fruit also improve sleep quality.[71]

Beware!

The old wives tale is true, **blue cheese** gives you weird dreams.[72]

Just like the caffeine in tea and coffee, **nicotine** wakes you up. You wouldn't drink a coffee before bed, so don't smoke either. Smoking **4 hours** before bedtime can disrupt your sleep.[73]

If you have trouble sleeping, try these tips...

- Do your exercise in the **morning.** People say that it helps them to sleep.

- **Set an alarm** to remind you to go to bed.

- **Don't medicate!** Just like alcohol, sleep medication gives the impression that you sleep better because you fall asleep quicker, but the quality of your sleep is worse.[74]

- If you can, take medications in the **morning** because medication can mess with your sleep.[75]

- Take a **hot** bath or shower before bedtime.[76]

- Live by the **3pm** rule. Don't nap or drink caffeine after 3pm.

- Turn down the heating. You sleep better in a **cool room.**[77]

- Use **black-out** curtains. Even a small amount of light can disrupt your sleep.[78]

- Don't **watch the clock.** Take all clocks out of the room. Put your phone out of reach where you can't check the time. If you are lying awake, put your earphones in. Listen to some relaxing music or a meditation track until you feel sleepy again. There's nothing like meditation to make you sleepy! Open an audible account and download a meditation track as your free gift.

- Stop watching **screens** at least an hour before you sleep.[79] The light from screens worsens your sleep quality.[80] You fall asleep quicker if you read a paper book or listen to an audiobook.

Bottom Line

Quality sleep prevents dementia.

NICOTINE IS GOOD FOR YOU BUT VAPING ISN'T

The problem is breathing vapour into your lungs.

Nicotine has been around for centuries. Most classic art and literature were powered by nicotine. Nicotine helps your **brain.** It's a stimulant, like coffee. Without tobacco, nicotine is fabulous for an ageing brain. It protects against brain **diseases** like Parkinson's and Alzheimer's.[81] Nicotine helps your **focus, memory,** and **fine motor skills.**[82]

Like smoking, vaping inflames your lungs which puts you at risk of infection.[83] Vapers are...

- 34% more likely to have a **heart attack**
- 25% more likely to develop coronary **artery disease**
- 55% more likely to suffer from **depression and anxiety**[84]

Switch from vaping to one of these methods...

- Chew nicotine gum
- Put on a patch or cut it in half
- Spray nicotine in your mouth
- Chew on a nicotine toothpick

Buy online or in a pharmacy.

Biohackers use these methods to help their brain. They don't mind being addicted to a substance that is good for them. We are all addicted to caffeine after all! This is called "micro-dosing". For more information, read Dave Asprey's biohacking books.

Beware!

People under 25 shouldn't touch nicotine. The human brain is not **fully wired** up until 25 years of age.[85]

Bottom Line

If you smoke or vape, you don't have to give up nicotine.

Access the workbook - Health Hacker 30 Day Challenge - ***Avoiding Alzheimer's.*** *Start your brain fitness journey today!*

HEALTHY, HAPPY, HORNY

Sex makes you live longer.

Give your brain, body, and relationship a boost...

- The more sex you have, the more salivary immunoglobulin A (IgA) you have.[1] The more IgA you have, the **less likely** you are to become ill.
- You **sleep better** after orgasm.[2]
- An orgasm can cure a headache,[3] so you can't use that excuse any more! It also reduces childbirth pain—at a home birth, I suppose.[4] Endorphins and oxytocin are **pain-killing hormones** released when you have sex or masturbate.[5] [6]
- Sex releases growth hormone, which helps you **look young.**[7]
- A man who has had a heart attack **lives longer** if he has regular sex,[8] because it makes him fitter.
- Sex is **moderate-intensity** exercise, more than walking but less than jogging.[9] Men burn around 100 calories and women 69. What an appropriate number!
- Regular sex helps **weight loss.** The oxytocin hormone is the one that makes you feel all warm and fuzzy. It also helps to break down fat![10] It's especially good for **diabetics,** because it helps you to re-sensitise to insulin.
- Oxytocin lowers your **blood pressure.**[11]
- Orgasms boost your **immune system.** — SEE CORONAVIRUS

Tip!

If you are diabetic or have high blood pressure, tell your partner that sex is part of your rehabilitation.

ERECTILE DYSFUNCTION

Men who ejaculate often live much longer than those who don't.[12]

I guess they have something to live for….

The more you ejaculate, the less likely you are to develop **prostate cancer.**[13]

A fit penis is attached to a **fit body.** If you eat right, exercise, and are not too stressed, your penis should work just fine. Men who eat the **Mediterranean diet** have less difficulty getting it up.[14] The Mediterranean diet includes lots of vegetables and fruit, some fish and meat. They eat a **little** dairy and wheat. They drink some wine and use quality fat such as olive oil and butter.

<u>Exercise</u>

6 months of aerobic exercise could sort you out. Aerobic exercise is the type that leaves you **out of breath.** Do a minimum of 3 sessions of 35 minutes per week.[15]

- Exercise increases **testosterone**, which makes you hard.[16]

- **Losing weight** also increases testosterone, but exercise increases it more.[17]

- **Interval training** increases testosterone the most. This is where you go really fast and get out of breath.[18] - SEE HIIT

- Mix it up, because **lifting weights** also boosts testosterone.[19]

147

Tip!

Do you know how to test whether your lady partner was faking it or not? Check her chest to see if it's flushed with pink blotches. That's the orgasm flush. I suppose this only works with white women…

Pelvic Floor Exercises

Not just for women.

Men get **harder** and last **longer** when they train their pelvic floor. If your pelvic floor is toned, your penis works better. A strong pelvic floor pumps blood to the penis, making it harder. Squeeze the muscle you use to stop yourself having a piss; hold it for a few seconds, and release. Do this **20 times** a day. After three months, you should be able to get harder[20] and last longer in bed.[21]

Tip!

To make the habit stick, do it at a particular time of the day. This could be in the shower or brushing your teeth. The activity acts as a trigger, reminding you to do the exercise.

Bottom Line

The harder you work out and the more vegetables you eat, the harder your penis will be.

THE FEMALE ORGASM

Women who orgasm throughout their lives live longer.[22]

Orgasms are **cardio** for the brain. When you orgasm, your brain is flooded with **oxygen**. This is fantastic for the brain. If you have poor blood flow to the brain, you are more likely to develop **dementia.**[23] Only a **quarter** of women reliably orgasm when they have sex.[24] This is partly because women tend to **value** their partner's orgasms more than their own.[25] Could this be why **more women** develop dementia than men? Regular orgasms are also good for your **mental health.**[26]

Make pleasure your **priority** and exploit your body to its full health potential. It's never too late to start. Sexual satisfaction **increases** with age, but a third of older women suffer from low libido. Half of women over 80 are sexually satisfied, whether they have a partner or not![27]

Science is dominated by men. We know more about the stars than we do about the female orgasm. Yet, the main reason why women can't orgasm is because they don't know **how.**

First, a biology lesson...

Your legs are for walking, your eyes for seeing, and your **clitoris is for coming.**

All orgasms stem from the **clitoris.** Nerves originate in the clitoris and branch out through the vagina and the anus. Yes, women can have anal orgasms. The G-spot is a **map.** Visualise the stump of the G as the clitoris (the flat -). The top end of the C is the G-spot, It curves round the front vaginal wall behind the clitoris. The closer you get to it, the more intense the pleasure.

One study found that **37%** of women must touch their clitoris to reach orgasm. Just **18%** can orgasm vaginally.[28] Another study found that **75%** can only orgasm with the help of a vibrator, hands, or a tongue. **10 to 15%** percent never orgasm under any circumstances.[29]

Rubbing or vibrating your clitoris while having sex leads to a **super-orgasm.** If you know how to masturbate, you will be able to have a super-orgasm without a vibrator. If not, a small vibrator will be **easier.** Some positions lend themselves to this better than others. Start with spooning. You will know when you've come, because your vaginal muscles will contract and **spasm** for a while.

You must put the work in, too! The more you **move your pelvis**, the more chance you have of achieving a vaginal orgasm.[30]

Tip!

Try the less sticky, water-based lubrication. Order online.

Multiple Orgasms

All women can have multiple orgasms. For some it comes easy and for others it comes hard—no pun intended! While a man's brain shuts down after orgasm, a woman's **lights up.** They might feel like aftershocks, or they might feel as strong as the first. However, only 47% of women have experienced multiple orgasms.[31]

Our orgasmic potential is an evolutionary mechanism which ensured fertilisation. In our tribal period of human history, we used to have many sexual partners. It didn't matter who the father was. The whole tribe worked as one unit, looking after everybody's kids. Basically, tribes had orgies.

Tip!

If you want multiple orgasms, **change tempo** and technique. After the first, your partner should slow down and work back up to a **crescendo.** If you want a super-orgasm, use a vibrator on your clitoris or touch yourself.

Super-Orgasmic Women

Super-orgasmic women orgasm over and over again on a loop. 10 or 20 orgasms would be normal for them to achieve in one session. Their brains release a lot of a hormone called **oxytocin.** That's the hormone that makes you feel warm and relaxed. The more **turned on** you are, the more oxytocin your brain releases, and the **easier** it is to reach orgasm. Women who get turned on easily are more likely to be super-orgasmic.[32]

However, some can't reach orgasm through sex for many years, until they relax and experiment with a like-minded partner. Reaching orgasm is as much psychological as it is physical. To increase your orgasmic potential though the mind, look out for my upcoming—no pun intended— book…. MIND YOUR HEALTH

Super-orgasmic women all have one thing in common; they masturbate **alone.**

Masturbation

If you can't give yourself an orgasm, how can you **expect** someone else to?

You can't expect to have a beautiful garden without putting in the groundwork. In the same way, you can't expect to have a fantastic sex life if you don't know how to masturbate. **94%** of women have masturbated before.[33] While you're there, test the multi-orgasm theory— that **all women** are multi-orgasmic. They will likely be less intense than the first, but see if you can have two, or three, or four…

With food, the more you eat, the more you want to eat. In the same way, the more orgasms you have, the more you want to have.

Beware!

Masturbate yourself manually on occasion. It's not a good idea to rely solely on a vibrator. I have heard reports of women needing an increasing amount of stimulation to reach orgasm. In this case, your partner will likely feel sidelined. Plus, what would you do if the charge ran out? Become incredibly frustrated I imagine….

Pelvic Floor Exercises

A strong pelvic floor can pump more blood to your vagina, which makes you orgasm harder. Squeeze the muscle that you use to stop yourself from having a pee. Hold it for a few seconds and release, at least **20 times** a day. Yoga and Pilates also strengthen these muscles. You use the **same muscles** when you have sex. The more you have sex, the **stronger** the muscles and the **better orgasms** you will have.[34] To make the habit stick, do pelvic floor exercises at a particular time. It could be in the shower, or when you are drinking your first cup or tea in the morning. The activity acts as a **trigger** to remind you to do your exercises.

Vibrators were invented for two reasons; a) to treat female "hysteria", and b) to strengthen the **pelvic floor.** If you have incontinence, instead of ordering one of those contraptions you put up your vagina and squeeze, why not use a vibrator instead? Then you can work out your pelvic floor and your brain at the same time! You also have the added bonus of jumpstarting your libido.

Tip!

Make sure to get the one with **clitoral stimulation.** And don't worry about the neighbours finding out, the packaging is discrete. Else go to a sex shop. Just imagine the look on your partner's face as you walk into the shop together…

Change Your Lifestyle

As your **weight increases**, your **libido decreases.**[35] If you eat a lot of fried food and sugar, you develop bad cholesterol. The worse your **cholesterol**, the worse your sex life.[36] SEE - CHOLESTEROL, PRESCRIPTION MEDICATIONS

The **Mediterranean diet** makes you hornier.[37] Those Spaniards must be so randy!

Tip!

Let your orgasmic potential be your motivation. Next time you are trying to resist a sweet temptation, think about your orgasms.

<u>Exercise</u>

Just like men, women can't orgasm if they don't have enough **testosterone.** This is one of the reasons why hormone replacement therapy (HRT) increases libido.[38] **Muscle strengthening** training works best for women to increase testosterone.[39] - SEE EXERCISE

Tip!

Get a **hot** personal trainer. Then you can have someone to fantasise about whilst doing your dementia-preventing homework. No ladies, that does **not** count as cheating….

Bottom Line

For mind-blowing orgasms, look after your body, keep an open mind, and be willing to experiment. Practice makes perfect, and it's good for your health, after all.

THE CONTRACEPTIVE PILL

Shrinks your brain and your libido.

The contraceptive pill is the most common birth-control method, and the most likely to mess you up. It messes with your **hormones.** When you mess with your hormones, you mess with your brain, body, and your sex life.

- The contraceptive pill shrinks the hypothalamus part of your brain.[40] This affects your temperature, mood, appetite, sex drive, sleep cycles, and heart rate. The smaller your hypothalamus, the **sadder** and **angrier** you tend to be.

- Taking the pill makes you do **worse on tests.**[41]

- Women on the pill are more likely to be **depressed,**[42] and depressed people tend to be less sexually active.

- It can stop you **responding to therapy.**[43]

- If you are overweight, it puts you at risk of **a stroke.**[44]

- The pill can **inflame your gut.**[45]

- It can lower your **sex drive** and even make sex **painful.**[46]

Bottom Line

The pill makes you dumb, depressed, and unsexy. This is not a medicine—it's a nightmare! Ask your doctor about a non-hormonal contraceptive like the copper IUD.

Access the workbook - Health Hacker 30 Day Challenge - ***HEALTHY, HAPPY, HORNY.*** *Start your brain fitness journey today!*

BEAT YOUR ILLNESS

DEPRESSION & ANXIETY

Read this before you take antidepressants.

The uncomfortable truth is that we have **no real idea** how the brain works. The cause of depression is a **complex** mix of psychology and physiology. We know that genes play a part. Yet, you may never develop depression if nothing happens to trigger it. This could be a real-life experience or body-wide inflammation, which originates in the gut.

Depression can be so severe that you lose the ability to feel anything at all, not even sadness. There is **no way** a pill can fix that. Until you combat the cause, you will always suffer. **Get some therapy.** Don't waste time on the national health service waiting list. Find a therapist online on Betterwell, Talkspace or Amwell.

Changing your lifestyle can do **more** for depression than anti-depressants. It's more difficult than taking a pill—that's for sure! But it's so **difficult** to come off antidepressants once you start taking them; it's best to try another way to feel better first.

Eat Right

The gut and the brain are **linked.** If you eat food that your gut doesn't like, it becomes **inflamed.** This inflammation can spread around your whole body. Besides having a bad diet, **poor sleep,** and **stress** inflame you even more. People with poor mental health tend to have **more** body-wide inflammation than stable people.[1] Inflammation **triggers** depression and anxiety. It also makes you **feel worse** if you already have it. We know this because depressed people feel better **after** taking anti-inflammatory drugs.[2]

People with poor mental health tend to eat **more junk** food and **less fresh** food.[3] Likewise, people who eat **less sugar** tend to be happier.[4] If you eat too much sugar, chemicals in your brain become imbalanced. If this happens, you can become anxious.[5] People with poor mental health **feel better** when they cut out sugary snacks.[6] If you want to feel some immediate relief, cut out **carbohydrates** such as bread, potatoes, rice, and pasta. - SEE THE ONE AND ONLY CRASH DIET At least give up the most inflammatory food. - SEE JUNK FOOD JUNK YOU, ALCOHOL, DITCH THE MILK

To summarise, eating unhealthily causes inflammation, which triggers depression **if** you have the genes for it. Junk food is more likely to affect the mental health of someone who has depression in their family. While sugar is not toxic for most people, it's **poison** for depressed and anxious people.[7]

Antidepressants can make you feel **worse** in the following ways…

- They mess with your **sleep.**[8] Depression and sleep are **linked.** The more depressed you are, the worse you sleep. The worse you sleep, the more depressed you are.[9] - SEE SLEEP
- They mess with your **gut,**[10] which can worsen depression. Depressed people's guts are different from those of happy people. Depressed people tend to **lack** the bacteria strains "Coprococcus" and "Dialister".[11] The gut and the brain are linked. If your gut is unhappy, you are unhappy.

To fix your gut, see - GET THAT GUT FEELING

Instead of taking antidepressants, do some **exercise.** Exercise can prevent depression.[12] - SEE EXERCISE

Even **walking** for half an hour a day reduces depression.[13] Anxious people don't tend to exercise,[14] but high intensity exercise really **helps** them.[15] - SEE HIIT

Tip!

Antidepressants work because of the **placebo effect.** You think a pill is going to make you happy, so it makes you happy.[16] It's a self-fulfilling prophesy. Doing exercise can also have the **placebo effect.** Science says that doing regular exercise will make you feel better. You believe that it will make you feel better, so it does. You will also feel healthier, which will make you even happier!

<u>Supplements</u>

You might have a chemical imbalance which is making you feel even worse. Depending on the particular imbalance you have, different supplements work for different people. Experiment until you feel an improvement.

- **Magnesium** helps your body deal with stress.[17]
- **L-Tyrosine** helps your neurotransmitters to keep you happy and focused[18] and think clearly when stressed.[19]
- Take a **multi-B** vitamin.[20]
- And **St John's Wart**[21]

Tip!

Get daily **sunshine.** Sunshine makes you happy. If can't get sunshine, take vitamin D3 and get a an infra-red light.[22] — SEE RED LIGHT THERAPY

Bottom Line

Eating a healthy diet, doing regular exercise and getting sunshine will make you happier than taking anti-depressants.

Access the workbook - Health Hacker 30 Day Challenge - ***FEEL HAPPIER.*** *Start your happiness journey today!*

REVERSING TYPE 2 DIABETES

Reverse diabetes to save your brain.

When you eat or drink something sweet, your body releases **insulin**. This insulin gets the sugar out of your bloodstream. If you didn't, you would become dizzy from dangerously high blood-sugar levels.[23] **Carbohydrates** get broken down into sugar in your body. - SEE SUGAR You also need insulin to remove this sugar too. Excess sugar turns to fat. If you have too much fat, it spills out into your liver and stops it from producing insulin.[24] If you stop producing insulin, you have to inject yourself with it. If you **lose fat**, your pancreas starts to **produce insulin again.** Slim people can be diabetic too. It depends on how much fat is around your organs.

Why should I bother?

Diabetes damages your blood vessels so less blood is pumped to the brain. If you have diabetes you are more likely to get **depressed**,[25] suffer mental health conditions like **schizophrenia**,[26] and brain diseases like **Alzheimers.**[27] In fact, having type 2 diabetes **doubles** the risk of developing Alzheimer's.[28] You are also more likely to develop **cancer**,[29] especially colon cancer.[30] That's because your colon has a difficult task processing refined carbohydrates. - SEE JUNK FOOD

So how can I reverse it?

Regular **exercise** prevents and helps to reverse diabetes. **Weight training** controls blood sugar by pushing sugar into muscles.[31] - SEE EXERCISE

To start with, lift a weight 20 to 30 times. Take a 1-minute rest, and do it again. Every time you switch from one machine to another, work a different muscle group. The **heavier** you lift, **the better** your blood sugar control. But even lifting light weights will help.[32]

To get even better sugar control, train in a **fasted state.**[33] Drink your coffee or tea black before you go to the gym in the morning. **Combine** weight training and aerobic exercise. Aerobic exercise can lower your blood sugar for **3 days.**[34] You must work damn hard, though. The more out of breath you become, the better your blood sugar control. - SEE HIIT

A 20-minute walk **after a meal** lowers blood sugar,[35] as does **standing up.**[36] — SEE STAND UP FOR YOURSELF

To lower your blood sugar by 11% after a meal, alternate between standing and sitting. If you forget, set an alarm to sound every 30 minutes. Order a stand-up desk or make one yourself. I put my laptop on top of a box on my desk.

Tip!

Buy an exercise bike. You can have an excellent work out in just **12 minutes**. - SEE USE YOUR HEART RATE

What should I eat?

Refined carbohydrates and sugar **causes** diabetes. If you are concerned about developing diabetes, **reduce carbohydrates** such as bread, pasta, rice, cereal, and potatoes. Replace them with quality protein, good fat, and vegetables.[37]

Understand how your blood sugar works. Fruit juice is **as bad** for your blood sugar as fizzy drinks. - SEE SUGAR

The Quickest Reversal

Half of people who follow a **replacement meal** diet for a year reverse their diabetes.[38] If you reverse your diabetes, you will suffer far fewer health conditions than you otherwise would have done. In the UK, Nuut and Huel are the market leaders. They are nutritionally complete, so you don't have to worry about getting your vitamins and minerals. You will also save a lot of money!

If that doesn't sound appealing, try intermittent fasting or the Ketogenic diet. - SEE WEIGHT-LOSS

Tip!

If you are on diabetes medication, make sure it's the one that's good for you. Metformin tackles diabetes though the gut. Your gut bacteria actually **like** this drug.[39] Metformin can make you **live longer.**[40] It helps your **heart,**[41] and can **prevent cancer.**[42] Don't take **Rosiglitazone**. It can give you heart failure.[43]

Diabetes Supplements

Take these if you are overweight to prevent diabetes, or to help reverse it.

- **Berberine** is a Chinese herb that has been used to treat diabetes for thousands of years. It's **as good** as some diabetes drugs in controlling your blood sugar.[44] Take 1,500 mg per day (three doses of 500mg) before meals.

- **Fenugreek seeds** also control blood sugar.[45] Take no more than two teaspoons daily.

- **Moringa leaf** treats diabetes and dementia.[46] Buy Moringa powder online. Add it to green smoothies, soups, and stews. It tastes a bit like asparagus.

- **Cranberry extract** tackles diabetes through the gut.[47] It can also prevent urinary tract infections— unlike cranberry juice.

My Promise

Once you start to notice how much **energy** you have, how **clear** your thoughts are, how your aches and pains start to **fade away**—you will **want** to live a healthy lifestyle, and that's a promise!

Bottom Line

The less refined carbohydrates and sugar you eat, the less likely you are to develop diabetes. To reverse diabetes, cut them out of your diet. Exercise and supplements will speed up the process.

Access the workbook - Health Hacker 30 Day Challenge - **REVERSING TYPE 2 DIABETES.** *Start your journey to great health today!*

ARTHRITIS

Don't want to develop arthritis? Move to Spain!

Arthritis is the fastest growing cause of disability worldwide.[48] There are two kinds, **osteoarthritis** and **rheumatoid** arthritis. Osteoarthritis is the most common.[49] While osteoarthritis is caused by wear and tear over time, rheumatoid arthritis is an autoimmune disease. In this case, your immune system thinks that the soft tissue around the joints is a virus and attacks it. This causes fluid build-up, swelling, and pain.

What's to blame?

Having the genes for arthritis doesn't mean that you will get it. It depends on **what you eat.**[50] Overweight people are **more likely** to develop arthritis.[51]

A good diet can **prevent** rheumatoid arthritis. Eat **good fats** such as butter, dark chocolate, fatty fish, and coconut oil. And avoid refined **sugar!**[52] It's also a good idea to **avoid** anything that doesn't agree with you. - SEE INTOLERANCES

Relieving Symptoms

If you want to reduce the pain, you must **tackle the cause**—the inflammation.

An anti-inflammatory diet is full of fibre and fresh produce with limited animal products.[53] Patients with osteoarthritis feel **less pain** after eating the Mediterranean diet for two weeks.[54] The

Mediterranean diet is packed with anti-inflammatory foods such as vegetables, fruits, whole grains, fish, and olive oil. Mediterranean people eat nuts and drink some wine. They eat little red meat, sugar, and dairy. To help your joints, eat **fatty fish** such as mackerel and sardines.

Try these pain busting tips...

- Take fish oil capsules. Only buy mercury free. Order online or ask in a health food shop.

- Lose weight. Being overweight makes the pain worse.

- Take **potassium**.[55] - SEE POTASSIUM

- Do some exercise! **87%** of osteoarthritis patients say it reduces their pain.[56] - SEE EXERCISE

- Avoid junk food. — SEE JUNK FOOD JUNK YOU

- Avoid inflammatory red meat and milk. - SEE DITCH THE MILK

- Submerse your fingers in ice-cold water. — SEE CRYOTHERAPY

- Use an infrared lamp on your joints — SEE RED LIGHT THERAPY

Bottom Line

If you don't want to get arthritis, eat fresh food and avoid junk food. If you have arthritis already, go to Spain to see how they eat. What a good excuse!

*Access the workbook - Health Hacker 30 Day Challenge – **ARTHRITIS** Start your journey to happy joints today!*

SINUS PROBLEMS

Tackle the cause, not the symptom.

15% of the UK population have sinusitis. The UK healthcare system spends more than £100 million annually on treatment.[57] Sinusitis occurs when your nasal passages become inflamed and blocked. If you are always blowing your nose and feel **pressure** in your sinuses, you have sinusitis. It can become painful and you can lose your sense of smell.

What causes sinusitis?

Many things can cause it, so it's **tricky** to treat. Chronic sinusitis lasts at least 3 months, whereas acute lasts less than a month.

2% of cases are due to a bacterial infection which can be treated with antibiotics.[58] Sometimes, the antibiotics don't work because the bacteria can **hide away** in your nasal passage.[59] This makes it chronic. The only thing you can do is treat the symptoms.

For the rest of cases, you must tackle the **inflammation.** Perhaps your body doesn't like something that you put in it, or perhaps it's something in your environment. You have the task of **finding out** what it is.

It could be your diet…

Inflammatory food can inflame your sinuses. The typical **western diet** is inflammatory. Refined carbohydrates, too much red meat (especially cheap meat), sugar, milk, and alcohol can inflame you. - SEE JUNK FOOD JUNK YOU, DITCH THE MILK, ALCOHOL, INDUSTRIAL MEAT, SUGAR

The **Mediterranean diet** is anti-inflammatory. They eat vegetables, local fruits, whole grains, fish, olive oil, nuts, and drink some wine. They don't eat a lot of red meat, sugar, or dairy.

You could also suffer inflammation if you're intolerant to something. — SEE INTOLERANCES

Inflammation **starts in the gut.** If you look after your gut, your gut looks after you. - SEE GET THAT GUT FEELING

Prebiotic and probiotic foods help some people with sinusitis.[60] - SEE PREBIOTICS AND PROBIOTICS

It could be candida...

Most sinus problems are caused by candida,[61] which is a **yeast overgrowth.** Other symptoms of a yeast overgrowth are being moody and tired. Antibiotics won't help because they target bacteria, not fungi.

If you want to test the theory, try this anti-candida program...

Step 1 - Stop drinking **alcohol** and **milk.** Stop eating refined **sugar** and starchy **carbohydrates** such as bread and pasta. If your sinuses get better, you may have found the cause.

Step 2 - Eat garlic, pomegranate, aloe vera, coconut oil, and turmeric. If your symptoms improve again, you know you have found the cause.

Step 3 - Go into a health shop and ask for probiotic supplements containing "lactobacillus". Otherwise, type "lactobacillus" into a search engine and order online.[62]

Step 4 - By an anti-candida diet book.

It could be an allergy...

Lastly, sinusitis could be caused by an **allergic reaction.**[63] If you have itchy eyes, it's probably an allergy. If taking anti-histamines makes your symptoms worse, it's not an allergy!

You want to find out what you are allergic to so that you can **avoid it.** Here are a few possibilities to try.

<u>**Histamine**</u>

Histamine is in **fermented foods** such as Kimche. If eating fermented foods make you worse, you have a histamine allergy. - SEE PROBIOTICS AND PREBIOTICS

Other histamine foodstuffs are vinegar, alcohol, aged cheese, dried fruit, avocados, eggplant, spinach, shellfish, and processed meat. Cut out these foods to see if it helps. If so, you have found the cause!

I feel bizarre when I eat Kimche. It makes my heart beat really fast. When you are sensitive to a food, your heart rate rises. Some symptoms of food sensitivities are bizarre. For example, I feel hot and sweaty when I eat a lot of vinegar.

If you identify a histamine sensitivity, type into a search engine "histamine food" to learn more about foods to avoid.

Chemicals

Chemicals can also affect your sinuses. A friend of mine had terrible sinus problems. When she got rid of her household cleaning products, her sniffles **disappeared.**

Stop using toxic cleaning products. — SEE CLEANING PRODUCTS

Make your own. Mix 1 cup baking soda, a squirt of washing up liquid, a tablespoon of white vinegar and ½ cup of water. Pour the liquid into a spray bottle and shake to mix.

If your sinuses get better, you know that you are sensitive to chemicals. You want to make your environment as **clean** as possible. — SEE AVOIDING TOXINS

Food Preservatives

Some people are allergic to the preservatives found in processed food and alcohol. To test this theory, eat nothing from a **packet or container** for two weeks. If this works for you, you will be on a forced natural diet for the rest of your life. Congratulations!

Treating the Symptoms

Nasal sprays don't work well.[64]

There's a new way to treat your sinuses without drugs! A **micro-current machine** relieves pain and congestion by sending pulses through your sinuses to relieve inflammation. Use it on your sinuses for five minutes to feel relief.[65] Buy "ClearUp" online for $149.00.

Do a nasal **breathing exercise** every day.[66] Type into YouTube "Luna Pranayama" to learn how.

Tip!

Do some **exercise.** Exercise decreases inflammation, so it should help your sinuses. It seems counter-intuitive, but exercise clears the sinuses of allergy sufferers. - SEE EXERCISE, IBS AND ALLERGIC DISEASES

Bottom Line

Unless you are one of the 2% with a bacterial infection, your body is trying to tell you to change something. Keep trying new approaches until you find the cause, and cut it out the best you can.

Access the workbook - Health Hacker 30 Day Challenge - **SINUS PROBLEMS.** *Start your journey to happy sinuses today!*

IBS & ALLERGIC DISEASES

Discover how IBS, asthma, eczema, and allergies are linked.

Irritable Bowel Syndrome (IBS) is a common condition that affects the digestive system. It's usually a lifelong problem. It can give you stomach cramps, bloating, diarrhoea, and constipation. The symptoms tend to come and go. Milder symptoms are a rumbly tummy, farting, burping, heartburn, or a stomach ache.

Allergic diseases have dramatically increased over the last few decades. Examples include asthma, eczema, hay fever, anaphylaxis, and food allergies. We now know that they start in the gut.[67] People with an irritable bowel are **more likely** to develop these allergic diseases.[68] Likewise, people with asthma are more likely to develop IBS.[69] The gut affects your **skin, respiratory** and **immune system.** If allergic diseases start in the gut, they can be **treated** via the gut.

The brain and gut are **linked.** If you have IBS, you are more likely to develop **mental health** problems such as anxiety.[70] The gut affects the brain, and the brain affects the gut. When you get anxious, you can feel it in your stomach. **Stress** aggravates IBS.

If you have IBS, it's in your interest to help your digestion the best you can. People with IBS are more likely to develop **cancer.**[71] **Polyphenols** in fruit, vegetables, coffee, tea, and dark chocolate fight cancer. - SEE POLYPHENOLS People with IBS have difficulty digesting food. If you **can't absorb** the nutrients from your food properly, you lose out on their cancer-fighting potential. Also, your gut controls your immune system. You need a fit immune system to fight cancer. Fix your gut, fix your immunity. — SEE GET THAT GUT FEELING

What causes IBS?

There are **many** causes. It could have been triggered by an event, or a combination of factors. For example…

-   You could have had an **infection** that messed up your gut bacteria.

-   You could have been born by **caesarean** section. Babies born by caesarean are more likely to develop IBS. Being covered in vaginal fluids at birth is important for your gut apparently![72]

-   You were fed poor quality food as a small child. — SEE GET THAT GUT FEELING

-   **Antibiotics** wipe out your gut bacteria. That increases your risk of developing IBS, allergies, and mental health problems.[73]

-   **Antacids** are medicines that suppress acid reflux. If a baby is given antacids or antibiotics, they are more likely to develop an **allergy** in childhood.[74]

Self-Medicating IBS

By treating the symptoms instead of the cause, you could be doing yourself **more harm** than good. Nearly 80% of IBS sufferers self-medicate, and a third of them do it wrong.[75] The most common medications are antacids for heartburn, laxatives, and anti-inflammatories. Taking antacids to relieve heartburn can make **bad**

bacteria grow in your gut,[76] which can cause stomach ulcers and cancer.[77] Laxatives and anti-inflammatories can also inflame your gut, especially if you take them over a long period of time. Don't treat the symptom, treat the **cause.**

Treating IBS & Allergic Diseases

IBS and allergic diseases can be helped via the gut. IBS sufferers have **fewer** gut bacteria, and the ones they do have are not well **balanced.** IBS and allergy sufferers have more strains of "Firmicutes" in their gut, the ones that make you fat.[78] People with IBS and children with asthma have **less** of the good bacteria "Bifidobacterium".[79]

Change Your Diet

If you have an allergic disease or IBS, feed your gut what it wants and avoid what it doesn't. Food or drinks that you are **sensitive** to can trigger symptoms. — SEE INTOLERANCES

Keep eliminating different foods until you find what works for you. People with IBS react to **different things.** Many react badly to milk, cheese, onion, cabbage, red meat, and alcohol (especially beer).[80] Try eliminating these first. Also, nearly half of people with IBS have the **gluten intolerance** gene.[81]

Most people try a diet called the LOW-FODMAP. This eliminates all **prebiotic** foods. The idea is to change the gut bacteria to make it healthier. This works for some people,[82] but not others. For some people, it makes their symptoms **worse.**[83] Research the diet online if you want to try it. But also take **probiotic supplements** to protect your gut bacteria.

The anti-inflammatory **Mediterranean diet** helps asthma sufferers. Eat fresh produce, fish, nuts, grains and good fats. Limit the dairy, red meat, alcohol and wheat.[84] **Eat slowly!** I used to eat quickly, and my stomach paid the price. Chew until it's mush in your mouth. You will have less difficulty digesting the food, so you will suffer less symptoms.

Tip!

If you have IBS, take **probiotic supplements.**[85] Multi-strain probiotics can improve your quality of life.[86] For best results, look for **10 billion** or more on the packaging.[87] Every gut is **unique**. Keep trying different strains of probiotics until you find the ones that work for you. Although it's not backed by research, probiotic supplements are worth a try if you have an allergic disease.

Eat Probiotic Food

As well as taking probiotic supplements, you want to eat the food that make good bacteria grow. "Bifidobacterium" and "Lactobacillus" help digestion. These bacteria live in **fermented foods.** Try live sauerkraut (not pasteurised), yoghurt, kimchi and miso. - SEE PROBIOTICS AND PREBIOTICS

"Clostridiales" and "Bacteroidetes" prevent children from developing asthma.[88] As does "Lactobacillus Rhamnosus".[89] You can find these bacteria in vegetables, peas, beans, whole grains, fruit and yoghurt. If any of these foods worsen your symptoms, **don't** eat them!

Tip!

Always buy **full-fat** yoghurt. The fat helps the good bacteria stick to your gut. Plus, saturated fat is the kind your brain likes. Get the **natural** version, and sweeten it with a natural extract like erythritol, raw honey, or fruit. Note that fruit and yoghurt is a difficult combination to digest.

Prebiotic Fibre

The gut is incredibly complex. Some people react well when they starve their guts of prebiotic fibre, like in the LOW-FODMAP diet. Others react in the completely **opposite way**. For some people, adding prebiotic fibre makes IBS better.[90]

Go into a health food shop and ask for prebiotic fibre powder, or order online. It will probably be labelled as INULIN.

Natural Remedies

The following natural remedies help IBS symptoms...[91]

- Take **peppermint oil** capsules and drink peppermint tea.
- Drink **aloe vera** juice or take supplements.
- Take a supplement form of the plant **Asafoetida.**

Tip!

Exercise helps IBS because it reduces inflammation.[92] Allergy sufferers particularly benefit from exercising in the cold.[93] - SEE EXERCISE

Bottom Line

IBS and allergic diseases can be helped via the gut. But there's no simple remedy because every gut is different. Try and try again until you feel relief.

Access the workbook - Health Hacker 30 Day Challenge - ***IBS & ALLERGIC DISEASES.*** *Start your health journey today!*

DODGE A BULLET

LOWER BACK PAIN

The most common disability worldwide.[1]

Taking anti-inflammatory drugs long-term is **bad** for your gut. If something is bad for your gut, it's bad for you. **Don't live your life in pain!** Try a few of these therapies. Different treatments work for different people.

- See a **physiotherapist.** If you are lucky, you might have a simple problem to fix. I used to suffer lower back pain, so I found a local physio online. He told me to strengthen my stomach muscles and to increase my back flexibility. As long as I work my core and stretch my back, I suffer no pain.

- **Aerobic** exercise reduces pain.[2] When you do aerobic exercise, more blood can reach the parts that hurt. This brings vital nutrients to heal the tissue. — SEE EXERCISE

- **Stabilisation** exercises reduce pain.[3] This is where you try to keep yourself stable. Ask a personal trainer to show you. Otherwise, type into YouTube "core stabilisation exercises" and follow the video.

- Correcting your **posture** reduces pain. Do 20 minutes stretching and posture correction exercises 3 times a week.[4] Ask a physiotherapist for instruction or type into YouTube "Posture correcting exercises".

- **Acupuncture** reduces pain. You will experience the most relief In the first few sessions.[5]

- **Hot and cold** therapy relieve pain.[6] Take a hot bath, or a dip in a British sea. Put a hot compress on your lower back or a pack of frozen peas. — SEE CRYOTHERAPY

- Try **red light** therapy. — SEE RED LIGHT THERAPY

Tip!

A medium-firm mattress is best for back pain.[7]

Preventing Pain

- **Tense** your stomach muscles when you lift something heavy.
- **Bend your knees**—not your back.
- Never lift in a **twisted** position.

The stronger your core and back, the less likely you are to hurt it. Work out your stomach muscles, stretch regularly, and do aerobic exercise.[8]

Tip!

If you hang off a bench to work your core, don't swing up and arch your back. Follow the advice of my chiropractor... "The worst thing you can do is to over-extend your back. Don't swing into any position that your back wouldn't normally be in." Simon - Pure Chiropractic Clinic - Staines Upon Thames, UK.

The 2-minute daily challenge!

Prevent back pain with two minutes a day!

- **The Plank** - Hold a push-up position, but don't actually drop all the way down and back up. You might only be able to hold the position for a few seconds to begin with. Do this every day. When you can hit a minute, you have a strong core. It's important not to dip your stomach or lift your bottom. Ask somebody to correct you. Otherwise, type into YouTube "Plank Posture" to watch a video. If your arms and wrists hurt, drop down to your elbows.

- **The Dead Hang** - Hang from an overhead bar. Install a pull up bar in the doorframe of your house. Jump up and hang from it for as long as you can. Do it once every day. When you can hold it for a minute, you are pretty strong! If you feel adventurous, you might want to try a pull up.

Bottom Line

You don't have to live in pain. Keep trying new approaches.

Access the workbook - Health Hacker 30 Day Challenge - **LOWER BACK PAIN.** *Start your health journey today!*

INFERTILITY

In the EU, 1 in 6 couples are infertile.

Male infertility is now the biggest cause.[9] Their health has declined in recent years, along with the quality of their sperm. These days, men are likely to be **unfit** and **infertile.**

An unhealthy lifestyle produces **free-radicals,**[10] which **damage** sperm. If your sperm gets damaged, your partner is more likely to **miscarry.**[11]

If you are trying for a baby…

- Eat plenty of **vegetables** and some **fruits.** You need a lot of antioxidants to fight free-radicals. — SEE POLYPHENOLS

- Eat **fatty fish** such as mackerel and take mercury free **fish oil.**[12]

- Wear a face mask if you work with **pesticides** or **anti-parasitics.** Men who work with these substances are more likely to have a premature baby. Babies born in the countryside are bigger than urban babies[13] — unless you live near a farm that sprays pesticides.[14]

- Cut down on **caffeine.** Some caffeine is good for you, but excessive intake **damages** sperm.[15] Besides coffee and tea, don't drink too many caffeinated fizzy drinks, especially **energy drinks.**[16] - SEE ENERGY DRINKS CAN KILL YOU

- Quit **smoking.** Smoking can ruin sperm.[17] — SEE NICOTINE IS GOOD FOR YOU BUT VAPING ISN'T

- **Exercise.** Exercise lowers stress, which helps your sperm.[18] Fit rats have more intelligent babies.[19] — SEE EXERCISE

The **good news** is that it only takes **two and a half months** to make new sperm. If you go on a health kick, you can improve your sperm almost immediately.[20]

IVF

Sometimes the problem is not with the sperm. The damage happens on the way out. Sperm taken from the **testicles** of an infertile man can be **as good** as sperm from a fertile man.[21] If you get IVF, pay the extra 10% and get the sperm taken straight out of the testes. Freeze it so you can use it again if the first round doesn't work.

Tip!

Vitamin D improves sperm.[22] Get daily sunshine on your skin and take D3. - SEE VITAMIN D

Bottom Line

You have the **power** to improve your sperm.

Women

If you are healthy before you get pregnant, you will have a healthier baby.[23]

Ideally, you will have a good diet, exercise regularly, not smoke or get drunk **before** getting pregnant. Your baby's skeleton and **bones** will suffer if you are pre-diabetic or diabetic.[24] - SEE REVERSING TYPE 2 DIABETES

Fertility tips…

- Women should take iron and folate **before** they get pregnant, not just during pregnancy.[25] - SEE IRON, FOLATE

- Some caffeine in tea and coffee is alright, but drink other **decaffeinated** drinks too.[26]

- Exercise **whilst** pregnant is good for your baby's bones,[27] and good for yours, too![28] - SEE EXERCISE

- **Try not to worry.** Stress during pregnancy can affect the health of your baby. Stress inflames your body, which can hurt the foetus.[29]

- People with **sleep apnoea** repeatedly stop breathing when they sleep. Women with this condition have smaller babies.[30] The main cause of sleep apnoea is being overweight. — SEE WEIGHT-LOSS

Bottom Line

Both you **and your partner** should live a healthy lifestyle while trying for a baby. Eat healthy meals and exercise together. If you didn't know, sex is exercise! - SEE HEALTHY, HAPPY, HORNY

*Access the workbook - Health Hacker 30 Day Challenge – **FERTILITY** Start your baby making journey today!*

BLUE LIGHT

It makes flies age quicker.[31]

Your phone, computer, and bright lights could be **ageing you** prematurely.

Blue wavelengths can damage **eye cells.** The worst lights are **fluorescent light**, such as strip lighting in an office.[32] **Flashing** lights and **LED** can also strain your eyes.

Don't think that you are protected from blue light just because you wear glasses with a blue tint; most only block around **15%** of screen light.[33] They have **no real effect** on sleep quality, eyestrain, or eye health.[34] The best strategy to avoid eye problems, is to reduce digital use.

To reduce blue light, try these tips:

- **Dim the screen** brightness on your tablet, computer, and phone.

- Wear yellow-tinted, **blue-blocking glasses** under artificial lights. You really notice how much your eyes are straining when you take them off. Order online.

- Install **dimmer switches** in your home. Make the lights dim enough that you can still see.

- Install **red lights.** Make your house a sexy boudoir! Also, red lights outside don't attract insects.[35]

- **Reduce screen time** by reading a paper book instead of an e-book.

Tip!

Blue light causes **wrinkles.**[36] Use a SPF moisturiser indoors.

Lutein is a supplement that protects your eyes from blue light.

Bottom Line

Simple changes to your habits and light fittings can massively reduce your exposure to blue light.

*Access the workbook - Health Hacker 30 Day Challenge - **BLUE LIGHT** Start your health journey today!*

CORONAVIRUS

Learn how to protect yourself from the next outbreak.

In the UK, 90% of people who died as a result of the 2020 Covid-19 outbreak had two or more **underlying** health conditions such as diabetes, obesity and heart disease. The Prime Minister of the UK, Boris Johnson, struggled to overcome the virus. He is convinced that being unfit and overweight caused him to be hospitalised.

Your immune system weakens as you age. That's why older people are more likely to be affected by viruses than young people. People who suffered the most severe symptoms were severely lacking T-cells. T-cells are responsible for clearing infection from the body. Simple lifestyle changes can **boost** your T-cells and **protect** your immune system.

- **Exercise** strengthens your immunity. Lifetime cyclists up to 79 years of age still have the immune systems of young people.[37] It's never too late to start! **Every session** strengthens your immunity. - SEE EXERCISE

- Don't wreck yourself with vodka. **Alcohol** might make you happy in the short term, but it can wreck your immunity.[38] If you feel the effects the next day, you have drunk too much! - SEE ALCOHOL

- Get quality **sleep.** Sleep boosts your immunity.[39] — SEE SLEEP

- Look after your **gut.** Your gut controls your immune system. If you have a happy gut, you have a good immune system.[40] The more junk you eat, the more likely you are to get sick. - SEE GET THAT GUT FEELING, JUNK FOOD JUNK YOU

- Chill out. When you **stress,** your immune system can't fight infection properly.[41]

- Take **prebiotic fibre powder.** It improves your immune system through your gut.[42]

- Drink **hibiscus tea.** Its antibacterial properties can prevent a cold or flu, and if you drink it while you have a cold, it speeds up your recovery time.[43] If you don't like tea, order hibiscus flower pills online.

- Get your flu jab in the **morning.** When elderly people get flu jabs, only half of them work. Morning flu jabs are more effective because your immune system works better in the morning, right after a good night's sleep.[44]

- Get some **sunshine.** Going out in the sun boosts your immunity. - SEE THE SUN IS YOUR FRIEND

- Have regular **orgasms**, with a partner or alone. Orgasms boost your immune system.[45] - SEE HEALTHY, HAPPY, HORNY

- Walk **barefoot.** - SEE GROUNDING

- Swim in a **cold** sea. - SEE CRYOTHERAPY

Bottom Line

Living a healthy lifestyle boosts your immunity.

Access the workbook - Health Hacker 30 Day Challenge - **UPGRADE YOUR IMMUNITY.** *Start your health journey today!*

GIVE BLOOD

Middle aged men who give blood are less likely to have a heart attack.[46]

Over time, iron is deposited in your organs, where it can cause problems. Too much iron in your blood makes it more likely that you will develop **breast cancer**[47] and **fatty liver disease.**[48] Donating blood **removes excess iron** from your bloodstream. I guess those 17th century doctors who used leeches were on to something!

Donating blood regularly lowers your **cholesterol** and prevents **heart problems**[49] because it removes the oxidants that damage cells. At the same time, it increases antioxidants which **fight cell damage.**[50]

You can burn **650 calories** per pint of blood donated, and you will be a pound lighter of course!

Beware!

Having too little iron is just **as bad** as having too much.

You lose a lot of iron when you menstruate. If you have periods and don't eat a lot of red meat, you should supplement with iron. — SEE IRON

Bottom Line

When you donate blood, you are not just helping someone in need, you are also be helping your health.

UPGRADE YOURSELF

FIX YOUR VISION

Think of your eyes as muscles. Exercise strengthens them.

Have you ever noticed that your eyes get worse when you start to wear glasses? That's because your eyes become lazy. Your vision **fluctuates,** sometimes it's better than at other times. If you wear glasses that are too strong, your vision worsens.

Tip 1 - Make your eyes work harder.

Get your eyes tested, but get the prescription made up a little weaker. Every time you are tested for new glasses, the prescriptions should get weaker.

Tip 2 - Read the small print.

Stick a page of small print to your kitchen cupboard or bathroom mirror. Read it without your glasses on when you are waiting for the kettle to boil or cleaning your teeth. You can print one off from the workbook - FIX YOUR VISION

Tip 3 - It's not just about the carrots.

A bad diet can make you **go blind.** If you don't eat the right nutrients, your **nervous system** gets damaged and you lose your sight.[1]

Avoid junk food. People who eat junk have more heart problems, more cancer and **worse vision.** — SEE JUNK FOOD JUNK YOU

Eat good fats, fresh vegetables, fruits, and nuts. By the way, peanuts are not nuts— they are legumes.

Tip 4 - Take Vitamins

Vitamins C, zinc, and **copper** stop your eyes degenerating.[2] You can get these together in one pill. Order online.

Lutein protects your eyes from the blue light that screens give off. As a side bonus, lutein helps your **brain.**[3] If you have trouble driving at night, take both Lutein and **Zeaxanthin,** and eat spinach.[4]

Tip 5 - Help Your Gut

Bad gut bacteria can trigger an autoimmune response. This is where your immune system attacks healthy cells, even those in your eyes.[5] **Glaucoma** is an autoimmune disease. It starts in the gut.[6] A **diverse** gut bacteria can prevent autoimmune disease.[7] - SEE GET THAT GUT FEELING

Tip 6 - Go Outside

Near-sightedness is a **global epidemic.** When my parents were at school, wearing glasses was the exception, not the norm. Nowadays, it seems as though every other child wears glasses. Kids play outside less and watch more screens, so they have worse eyesight. The more children **play outside**, the **less** near-sightedness they have.[8]

Tip 7 - Exercise

It prevents your eyes from degenerating.[9] - SEE EXERCISE

Tip 8 - Wear your sunglasses wisely.

To avoid cataracts, wear sunglasses in strong sunlight.[10] But don't wear them all the time, because natural light is good for your eyes and can help induce sleep.

Tip 9 - Protect them from screens.

Natural light is better for your eyes than artificial light. Work under a window whenever possible. You will have less eyestrain and headaches, and feel more alert.[11]

While working for long periods on a computer, take **stare breaks.** If you have nothing to gaze at outside, put a pot plant on your desk and gaze at it whenever you feel your eyes straining.

Use eye drops before a long stint working on your computer.

Tip 10 - Get the new Laser surgery.

If you mess up your eyes by looking at screens all day, you can get keyhole laser surgery. People who previously couldn't get laser surgery can now get it done. It's called **Relex Smile.** It's as good at treating near-sightedness as the old technology, with fewer side effects.[12]

Bottom Line

If you want to see your 100th birthday, eat healthy food and be kind to your eyes.

Access the workbook - Health Hacker 30 Day Challenge -
FIX YOUR VISION. *Start your journey to great vision today!*

A PERFECT SMILE

British people have a reputation for terrible teeth. If you are anything like me, you have weak teeth and a mouth full of silver fillings.

Hunter-gatherer tribes never failed to astound scientists with their perfect, white teeth. This was especially striking because they had no dentists! Their diet was perfect for teeth health. They ate **little sugar** and a lot of foods rich in **K2**, which fights tooth decay.[13] You can find K2 in **red meat, butter, eggs,** and **fermented soy.** I take a K2 supplement alongside D3, because they work together. Your teeth can't tell the difference between natural and refined sugar. To protect your teeth, eat fruit for **dessert** instead of a snack.

Beware!

Don't take calcium unless you are deficient. - SEE BEWARE OF CALCIUM

Tip!

See a **hygienist** regularly. They scrape off plaque and remove stains. They also tell you which teeth you are missing while brushing.

Oil Pulling

Oil pulling **detoxifies** the mouth. Swish a tablespoon of coconut or sesame oil in your mouth and go about your business for **10 - 20** minutes. The oil mixes with your saliva to make a cleaning liquid, which binds to the bacteria and plaque. It reduces inflammation, bad breath, and whitens your teeth. You will have healthier teeth if you do it regularly.[14] Make sure to **spit it out** and rinse your mouth with water. Leave the oil on your bathroom shelf to remind you, and hope that nobody talks to you while you have your mouth full!

Activated Charcoal

Health experts eat activated charcoal to **detox** their bodies. The **toxins** attach to the charcoal and eventually, go down the toilet. Once a week, wet your toothbrush and dip it in activated charcoal **powder.** Otherwise, a special toothbrush with charcoal bristles cleans your teeth better than a regular toothbrush.[15] Order online.

Chew Gum

Chewing special gum reverses tooth decay.

Chewing gum helps you to **focus,**[16] reduces **stress**[17] and even **burns calories.**[18] Smelling **peppermint** also reduces your **hunger** and **cravings.**[19]

Chewing gum after eating makes you produce saliva, which helps you to **clear away** bits of food.[20] Gum with sugar rots your teeth, and sugar-free gum has nasty artificial sweeteners. — SEE ARTIFICIAL SWEETENERS

Buy **xylitol** gum online. This gum is better than sugar-free at preventing tooth decay.[21] Xylitol is a natural sweetener found in fruit, vegetables, berries and wood. Chewing xylitol gum can **reduce** bad bacteria by 75%[22] and **reverse** dental cavities! Children who chew xylitol gum have fewer cavities than those who don't.[23] Chewing for

20 minutes after eating also **improves** your tooth enamel.[24] If you keep up the habit for 3 weeks you can **reduce** dental plaque.[25]

Avoid Mouthwash

It's a disgrace that mouthwash companies advertise on TV.

Mouthwash is to your mouth is what antibiotics are to your gut. Mouthwash kills both the good and bad bacteria in your mouth. You need good bacteria to **fight infection.**

Toothpaste has **more fluoride** in it than mouthwash. By using mouthwash after you brush, you **wash away** the protective fluoride. Also, some mouthwashes have a **low pH** level which erodes your teeth.[26]

It's hard to believe, but people who use mouthwash twice a day are more likely to develop **high blood pressure.**[27] That's because your mouth bacteria helps to release **nitric oxide.** By messing with your mouth bacteria, you mess with your ability to produce nitric oxide.

If you use mouthwash every day over a long period of time, you have a higher risk of developing **diabetes.**[28] It messes with the microorganisms in your mouth, which impacts your ability to metabolise sugar.

Just to top it off, mouthwash **stains** your teeth![29]

Mouthwash should only be used for a short period of time, and only if you have a **specific problem** such as gum disease.

Tip!

Using a tongue scraper twice a day after brushing **removes** bad bacteria that cause bad breath and decay.[30] It can even give you a more acute sense of **taste.**[31]

Bottom Line

Save the money you would spend on mouthwash to buy things that will actually help your teeth.

Access the workbook - Health Hacker 30 Day Challenge -
A PERFECT SMILE. Start your journey to beautiful teeth today!

THE SUN IS YOUR FRIEND

If you avoid the sun, you might die earlier than you should.[32]

Indoor living is a new lifestyle for humans. We used to spend the day hunting and gathering food. The sun is a **life-giving** energy force which offers major health benefits. These days, we are so afraid of getting skin cancer that we try to avoid it.

Of course, getting burnt is **awful** for your skin. Use sunscreen in strong sunlight, but not all the time! Sunscreens stop you from absorbing vitamin D.[33] To make matters worse, pollution can reduce the sunlight filtering through.[34] Even if you take vitamin D3, you should **still** go outside. The sun gives you health benefits that you **can't get** from a pill.

Sunshine makes you **happy.** When you get sunshine on your skin, your brain releases **pleasure hormones** called endorphins.[35] Your brain releases these hormones when you do something it likes, such as eating, doing exercise, and having sex.

Sunshine is good for your **heart.** Scientists often wondered why Australians had fewer heart problems than the British. Sunlight helps your body produce **nitric oxide.**[36] This encourages blood flow. People who enjoy more sunshine have fewer **heart problems, strokes,** and lower **blood pressure.**[37]

Sunshine helps you **lose weight.** Have you ever wondered why you gain weight in winter? 30 minutes of summer sun without sunscreen a week can stop you from becoming **obese.**[38] The sun **breaks down fat.**[39] The fat cells underneath your skin actually shrink.[40]

Sunshine helps your **immune system.** It energises your **T cells,** which boosts your immunity.[41] This can protect you from developing an **autoimmune disease.**[42] Examples of autoimmune diseases are rheumatoid arthritis, psoriasis, inflammatory bowel disease, multiple sclerosis, and asthma. These conditions occur when your immune system attacks healthy tissue by mistake.

Sunshine protects you from **cancer.** If you get regular sunshine, you have **less risk** of developing breast, colon, and prostate cancer.[43] The higher your vitamin D level, the less chance you have of developing breast cancer. — SEE VITAMIN D

Sunshine is good for your **brain.** The less you go outside, the quicker your brain **deteriorates.**[44]

The sun makes your brain **fire signals** that help your **memory** and **fine motor skills,** making you more agile.[45]

You might have heard that sunbathing causes wrinkles. That's because it can damage your skin's DNA.[46] Red light therapy is a sun machine, but it can penetrate the skin without damaging it. It can helps you to produce **collagen,** which you need to make skin. — SEE COLLAGEN, RED LIGHT THERAPY

Yet, people with skin conditions often notice that it **clears up** when they go in the sun. The doctor may tell you to sunbathe if you have a **skin condition** such as psoriasis, eczema, jaundice, or acne.[47] Thats because UV light decreases inflammation. People with skin conditions also benefit from red light therapy.

Sunshine helps you **sleep.** When you get daylight in your eyes in the morning, your sleep clock **resets** itself.[48] If you don't produce **melatonin** before bedtime, you don't feel sleepy. Morning daylight in your eyes helps production of melatonin in the evening. **15** minutes outside **without sunglasses** is enough. You only need to wear sunglasses when the sun is strong. In the UK, that's between 11am and 3pm. Contact lenses, glasses, sunglasses, and windows block the sun. If you wear glasses, get into the habit of looking over the top of them when walking outside.

Sunshine helps your **vision.** Don't put sunglasses on a child. Sunlight is important for their **eye development.** Kids who spend more time **outside** are less likely to need glasses for nearsightedness.[49]

Tip!

Don't look directly at the sun!

Bottom Line

As long as you don't regularly get burnt, the sun does far more good than harm.

Access the workbook - Health Hacker 30 Day Challenge -
HEAL YOURSELF. *Start your journey to fabulous health!*

HEALING

RED LIGHT THERAPY

The healing power of the sun in your living room.

The sun is wonderful for your health, and so is red light therapy. Sometimes, it's called red light, sometimes UV light, sometimes far-infrared. I will call it infrared light. It's a **sun machine**, and treats many conditions helped by sunshine.

Infrared light heals your body in the same way that it makes **plants grow**.[1] It **stimulates** the cells underneath your skin,[2] and gives them more **energy** to repair themselves. Whereas a laser damages the top layer of your skin, infrared light therapy doesn't.

It even helps to make **stem cells.** Stem cells are the holy grail of cells—the kind that can become anything you need in the body.[3]

How does infrared work?

When light shines on water, the chemical **structure changes.** It becomes more dense than ordinary water. The electrons in the water separate and give it an **antioxidant** effect that **protects** cells from damage.[4] It helps normal cells to **develop** while suppressing the abnormal ones.[5] When scientists use light to change the structure of water, plants grow **twice** as fast.[6] Scientists think that infrared light does the same to the liquid inside your body.

If you want infrared therapy, you have two options. Type into a search engine **infrared sauna** to find a clinic nearby. Otherwise, buy an infrared **machine** online. Do your research and buy a quality device.

Infrared light can help your illness…

- If your **immune system** attacks healthy cells by mistake, it can lead to autoimmune disease. Infrared reduces the **inflammation** that the immune system causes. This helps people with autoimmune diseases such as arthritis, psoriasis, irritable bowel disease, and multiple sclerosis.

- Infrared also improves the health of people with **diabetes, heart disease,** and chronic **kidney disease.**[7]

- Just like sunlight, infrared makes you produce more nitric oxide, which helps to create blood vessels.[8] This improves your blood **circulation.**[9]

- A month of using a portable infrared machine lowers **blood sugar.** Set a wavelength between 9,000-12,000 and 30 megawatts. Just once a week for 15 minutes can make a difference.[10]

- Infrared is wonderful for your **brain.** It can stop the progression of Alzheimer's and Parkinson's Disease.[11]

- Infrared therapy reduces **chronic pain.**[12]

- It makes **chemotherapy** and **radiotherapy** patients feel better.[13]

- Infrared light reduces your **stress** hormone, cortisol.[14] Too much cortisol can cause depression, anxiety, poor sleep, and poor digestion.

- Using infrared twice a week for 15 minutes makes depressed people **happier**. It increases the happy hormone serotonin and reduces cell damage.[15]

Infrared can heal you…

Infrared light causes your body to release an **anti-inflammatory** compound.

- Athletes use infrared light to **recover** from exercise. Set the temperature to 35 - 50°C.[16]

- It heals inflammatory conditions such as **tendonitis.**[17] Set it to 5.4 megawatts.

- Heal a **cold sore**. Use a wavelength of 1072 for 2 days, 3 times a day, for 3 minutes.[18]

- Infrared helps your **hair grow.** If you have alopecia, use a wavelength of 808.[19]

- It stimulates collagen and elastin, which make your **wrinkles** less noticeable. Use it twice a week for 12 - 25 minutes on a low wavelength such as 611–650. Up to 850 is fine.[20] Red light can penetrate the skin without damaging the skin's DNA.

- It improves the appearance of **scar** and **stretch marks.**[21]

- It heals **sun damaged** skin at a wavelength of between 633 and 830.

- Direct it onto your **psoriasis**[22] or **eczema.**[23]

Tip!

Even healthy people reap the benefits of red-light therapy. Get into the habit of using it every day for 15 minutes.

Beware!

Use them at the recommended doses. You can have too much of a good thing.

Bottom Line

Infrared therapy is safe, effective, and widely used.[24]

CRYOTHERAPY

Keeping animals cool makes them live a quarter of their lifespan longer.[25]

Refrigerate yourself to improve your shelf life! Keeping your body temperature cool **preserves** your body,[26] making you age better. Take cold showers, swim in cold water, and turn down the heating.

You can go to a cryotherapy clinic and step into a temperature below -100°C. Otherwise, you can just treat a certain body part. But anything less than 2 minutes won't work.[27]

What's the point?

- Cryotherapy prevents **cell damage.**[28]

- It helps your i**mmune system.**[29]

- It reduces **inflammation.**[30] It treats **any condition** caused or aggravated by inflammation. This could be a problem with an organ, your nervous system, skin, or throat.

- The reduction in inflammation **reduces pain.**

- Cryotherapy is more effective than traditional methods in treating **arthritis.**[31]

- If you have a **spine issue,** cryotherapy can help you to move around better.

- People with a **frozen shoulder** show more improvement with cryotherapy compared to other therapies.[32]

- 3 months of cryotherapy reduces **back pain** and helps you move around better.[33]

- Cryotherapy improves **athletic performance.** It reduces the pain and inflammation from strenuous exercise, allowing quicker recovery.[34]

- It also treats **mental health** problems. Besides reducing inflammation, cryotherapy helps depression and anxiety by increasing **happy hormones** called endorphins.[35] To learn more about the role of inflammation in mental health, see DEPRESSION AND ANXIETY

- Cryotherapy treats fatigue,[36] helping **fibromyalgia** sufferers to have a better quality of life.[37]

- Cryotherapy treats **diabetes.** Being cold changes your gut microbiome, allowing diabetics to become sensitive to insulin again.[38]

How can I do Cryo?

- Type "cryotherapy chamber" into a search engine to find a clinic in your area. The price is around £60 ($70) a session.

- Take a cold shower. At the end of your shower, turn the temperature right down and direct it on your chest and face. It will sure wake you up!

213

- Swim in cold water. Your brain releases endorphins which make your feel **euphoric.** Afterwards, you feel **clear headed** and have **more energy** than normal.

- To recover from strenuous exercise, take a bath with ice packs in it.

- Treat a specific area. If you have pain in your fingers, dip your hands in ice cold water.

Beware!

Build up slowly. I learnt this the hard way. I filled a bowl with ice, put a straw in my mouth and submersed my face. The first time I did it for 5 minutes, my skin felt fantastic! The second time, I held it for 15 minutes, and I kind of froze my face off. My skin had never looked so terrible!

Don't be an idiot like me. Start with 5 minutes, then increase by a **few minutes** until 15 minutes.

Bottom Line

Being cold is good for your health, so quit whining!

GROUNDING

Walking barefoot can heal you.

Healers have been walking barefoot for centuries. They weren't as crazy as they seemed.

If you know about quantum mechanics, you know that the universe works in **mysterious** ways. Some things that happen are **completely impossible** —far beyond our comprehension. To study quantum physics, you must let go of everything you think you know about science. The first rule is that **anything** is possible.

Open minded people benefit from grounding, otherwise known as earthing. When you walk barefoot, you absorb the earth's **electric current.** Electrons spread through your body and have a **healing** effect.

-   Grounding decreases **inflammation,** so it helps your **immune system** fight against disease.

-   Wounds **heal faster** when the body is grounded.[39]

-   Sleeping on a grounding mat reduces **pain** and **stress.**[40]

-   It makes your **heart beat** at a healthier rhythm and makes **blood flow** easier.[41]

-   It helps you to **recover** from strenuous exercise.[42]

To ground yourself, your **bare skin** must touch the ground. If you are lucky enough to live by the sea, walk barefoot on the sand. Do some yoga on the grass, or just lay down on it, placing your palms on the ground. Stay at least **15** minutes. For major health benefits, buy a grounding mat. This mat lies underneath your sheet and emits the same electrical current as the earth does.

Tip!

Grounding helps jet lag.

Bottom Line

Your body is a battery that requires routine recharging.

Access the workbook - Health Hacker 30 Day Challenge - **HEAL YOURSELF.** *Start your journey to fabulous health today!*

AVOIDING TOXINS

We are **guinea pigs** in this new modern world. In a hundred years, most of the chemicals we encounter will be **banned.**

We are **swimming** in toxins, and you can't rely on the government to keep you safe. It takes a **long time** to prove that a substance is toxic, and even **longer** for the government to do something about it.

You can prove an association between a toxin and harm quite easily. Chemicals stay in circulation until scientists can prove that the toxin **caused** the harm. This is a long and drawn out process. If a researcher suspects that a chemical is toxic, it would be very difficult to get ethical approval to test it on humans. Some products take a hundred years to prove toxic.

Lead is one of these products. Until 1978, lead was used in paint. Likewise, farming herbicides have taken 50 years to be proven toxic. Also, chemicals are mixed together, so it can be tricky to pinpoint which one (or ones) caused the harm.

Understand that it's not in companies' interests to protect you. They can **repeat** studies until they get the result they want. If a chemical is proven toxic, they tend to replace it with an equally toxic one. It then takes another decade to prove the toxicity of the new chemical.

There are simple things that we can do to reduce our exposure to harmful toxins. Small changes make a big difference. You might not want to throw away every toxic substance you own. But you might make the effort to buy natural products in the future. High-street pharmacies now stock natural beauty products such as the "Garnier Organic" range. The more natural products you buy, the more companies are likely to research natural alternatives to harmful chemicals. Use your **purchasing power.**

If you follow this advice, you can feel comfort in the knowledge that you are keeping yourself safe from a toxic environment.

CLEANING PRODUCTS

Cleaning products have hazardous chemicals in them.[1]

- Disinfectants can give you **asthma.** Health-care workers who use **disinfectants** are more likely to have breathing problems.[2]

- New parents who use many cleaning products **at home** are more likely to have an asthmatic child.[3] Besides, germs are **good** for children. Babies who suck dummies (pacifiers) that are allowed to fall on the floor have **less** allergies, asthma, and eczema.[4]

- Cleaners have more **lung problems** as they age. Retired cleaners find it harder to breathe than people who didn't clean for a living.[5]

- COPD is a lung condition that causes breathlessness. Nurses who **clean at work** at least once a week have **22%** more chance of developing COPD.[6]

If I were a cleaner, I would wear a **face mask.**

Tip!

Make your own cleaning product. Mix 1 cup baking soda, a squirt of washing up liquid, a tablespoon of white vinegar, and ½ cup of water. Pour the liquid into a spray bottle and shake.

Bottom Line

Don't stress about germs, stress about chemicals.

COOKING METHODS

The more fried food you eat, the earlier you will die.[7]

How you cook your food can make it super **healthy** or super **cancerous.**

Chargrilled meat is cancerous because overcooked meat releases toxins.[8] If you eat a lot of **roasted or barbecued** red meat, you have a higher risk of developing cancer[9] and heart disease.[10]

Marinate your meat in **ale** to prevent the damage.[11] Marinating your meat before cooking in unfiltered beer stops it from becoming cancerous.[12] **Rosemary, oregano,** and **thyme** further protect the meat.[13]

The **longer** you cook meat for, the **worse** it is for you.[14] Swap your slow cooker for a **pressure** cooker. It damages the meat less than other methods.[15] The same rule applies to fish. Fry lightly, steam or boil quickly.[16] Sushi is raw fish, remember! **Steam** your vegetables to preserve the nutrients. The **less** time you cook your veggies for, the **more** nutrients they retain.

Fried food is alright, provided you use the **right fat.** Use olive oil on a **low heat.**[17] This oil is easily damaged, so buy the ones in dark glass bottles. Only use extra-virgin to drizzle on vegetables. At **high heat,** use coconut oil, butter, or ghee. Don't fry the meat for too long![18]

Ditch the vegetable oil. You need a balance between omega-3 and omega-6 fats. Vegetable oils overdose you with omega-6 fats. — SEE GET FAT

Vegetable oil also affects your **thyroid,** which lowers your metabolism and can make you **fat.**[19] **Don't use** seed oil such as sunflower or canola oil, either. They have a low smoke point and release toxins easily.[20]

Escape The Waves

Don't be like my father, who cooks bacon in the microwave.

Microwaving meat shrinks it and can make it toxic.[21] Microwaving meat can also increase its **cholesterol** content.[22] Microwaving vegetables is the **worst** way to lock in vitamins. Steaming is the best.[23]

Try to limit microwave use to when you are reheating a dish. I recently lived in Taiwan. I didn't see a microwave the whole time I was there. They have electric steam pots instead. You plug it into the wall, put your food inside and press down a lever. Ten minutes later, the lever pops up and you have a well-heated dish.

Tip!

If you must cook vegetables win the microwave, don't add water. This prevents the nutrients from leaking out.[24]

Bottom Line

How you cook your food is **as important** as what you eat.

HEAVY METALS

Cheap, scratched cookware leak toxins into food.

Never buy cheap aluminium pans.[25] They are toxic!

Do you have a Teflon pan in your kitchen? Years ago, a chemical in non-stick pans was proven toxic and replaced with different coatings. A few years ago, researchers found out that the replacement coating was just as toxic as the old one![26] If you have a Teflon pan, don't put it in the dishwasher. As soon as it scratches, dump it!

Choose iron, titanium, copper, anodised aluminium, ceramic, or glass cookware.

Beware!

Iron pots leach iron into food. That's great if you don't eat a lot of red meat. But too much iron is terrible for your health. — SEE GIVE BLOOD

Bottom Line

Buy some decent cookware.

MERCURY IS FISHY

40% of human mercury exposure is from canned tuna.[27]

There's a lot of mercury in the sea. Most of it is because of air pollution. Mercury is **toxic.**[28] It **damages** your chromosomes, immune system, and heart.[29]

When we eat mercury, it gets trapped in our **liver.** Fish can't get rid of the mercury they eat either. The more fish they eat, the more mercury gets trapped in their livers.[30] The **bigger** and older the fish, the **more** mercury tends to be in it.[31]

People who eat a lot of **predatory fish** like pike and perch have **higher levels** of mercury in their bodies.[32] Avoid fish such as cod, swordfish, and tuna.[33] Upgrade tuna for **sardines.** They contain less mercury and far **more nutrients.** Instead of cod, choose **pollock** or **haddock.**

Beware!

If you are pregnant, be **extra careful** to eat small fish.[34]

Tip!

Make sure that the **fish oil** you buy is mercury free. Cold-pressed is best, because heat damages the oil.

Bottom Line

The health benefits far outweigh the risks of seafood, as long as you don't eat big fish.

MERCURY FILLINGS

If you are British, you probably have a filling made of mercury.

If you are like me, you have a mouth full of them!

Silver or "amalgam" fillings are being **phased out** of British dentistry. They are toxic! The EU **banned** mercury in dentistry in **2018**. The UK is no longer part of the EU, and we are still using it today.[35]

It has taken over 100 years to prove that mercury amalgam fillings are toxic—they actually **cause** harm. Mercury fillings can trigger dementia, fatigue, MS, and insomnia. It can also make you anxious and moody, and affect your memory.[36] The wide range of symptoms made it incredibly hard to prove.

Bottom Line

Spend the extra money and get a white filling, else you risk toxic mercury exposure.

BPA

BPA is found in the umbilical cords of 9 out of 10 pregnant women.[37]

BPA is a building block in **plastic,** also used to line food **cans** and **packaging.** In one survey, BPA was in the urine of **93%** of Americans.[38] Your job can expose you to BPA. **Painters** have a lot in their urine.[39] New research shows that BPA testing is **flawed.** The problem is **much worse** than we thought it was.[40]

The effects of BPA exposure can be passed down for **three generations.**[41] Studies show that people with **cancer** have more BPA in their urine than normal.[42] But there is **no smoking gun** that BPA causes cancer.

BPA **harms** both animals and humans. The strongest evidence is that BPA gives children **behavioural problems.**[43] I witnessed this first hand as a high-school teacher! Even at "safe" levels, BPA can impact a child's **brain development** and affect their **behaviour.**[44] Children who are exposed to a lot of BPA have more behavioural and **mental health** problems.[45]

Even at **minuscule levels**— under what the government deems safe— BPA affects the hormones in an **unborn** baby rat brain, and effects how their genes express themselves.[46] It makes their **sex hormones** act differently[47] and damages their **DNA.**[48] In one study, turtles that were exposed to BPA before birth displayed more feminine behaviours.[64]

My grandma says that men didn't act effeminately when she was younger. I wonder if it's because of BPA...

BPA can also...

- Harm your **gut.**[49] Your gut is of vital importance to your health and wellbeing. - SEE GET THAT GUT FEELING

- Mess with your **insulin.** If your insulin level is messed up, you are more likely to develop diabetes.[50]

- Make you put on **weight,** which puts extra pressure on your heart.[51]

- Predispose you to **diabetes.** Exposure to BPA increases the likelihood that children develop diabetes in later life.[52]

- Make female animals **infertile.**[53]

To avoid BPA...

- Reduce the food you buy in **plastic** or **canned** containers. This can make a real difference to your BPA levels.[54]

- Switch from canned to **frozen** food. If you eat from a can, **rinse** the BPA off the food before you eat it.

- Don't put plastic in the **dishwasher** or **microwave.**

- Don't put **boiling water** into plastic cups or containers.

Beware!

You can't trust "BPA-Free" products.

The evidence against BPA was too great to ignore. Companies replaced BPA with BPS, which was even worse than BPA! BPS messes with your **heart.**[55] Just like BPA, the damage passes from generation to generation.[56]

Bottom Line

BPA is nature's way of telling you not to be lazy. Cook your child fresh food, else they might start climbing the walls.

PERSONAL CARE PRODUCTS

While cancer rates in men are decreasing, they remain stable for women.

Humans love to put chemicals on themselves in the name of fashion. In Victorian England, aristocrats would slather lead-based paints on their faces to make themselves whiter.

Countries ban different products. While some countries have banned 1,400, the US has only banned **9**.[57] In 2016, Johnson & Johnson were fined $324 million. They **knew** that their talcum powder had cancerous chemicals in it. They continued to sell it to customers, who then developed cancer.[58]

The **EWG** have been monitoring chemicals in beauty products for over a decade. They say that chemicals are to **blame** for many cases of cancer, infertility, allergies, thyroid conditions, diabetes, and ADHD.

Cancer rates are in decline, **apart from** thyroid, liver, and skin cancer. These cancer rates are **rising.** Meanwhile, the incidence of cancer in men is **decreasing,** but the amount of women who develop cancer remains **stable**.[59] What do women do that men don't? Slather beauty products all over themselves! Women who **dye their hair** are more prone to breast **cancer** than those who don't.[60]

The fact that people who use beauty products develop more cancer is **not proof** enough to ban them. There are so many chemicals in each product that it's virtually **impossible to track** which one—or ones—caused the illness. Industry groups say that these chemicals at small doses are safe; but we use a **variety of products**, so the doses aren't that small! The damage is likely caused by a **combination** of chemicals over time.

The EWG advise that we avoid the following chemicals in personal care products:

- **Formaldehyde** in keratin hair treatments, body soap, and nail polish.

- **Triclosan** is most commonly found in toothpaste, mouthwash and anti-bacterial hand gels. It is easily absorbed and impact your gut. — SEE GET THAT GUT FEELING

- **Coal tar** in hair dyes and shampoos.

- **Heavy metals** such as lead in lipsticks, hair dyes, and clay products.

- **Teflon,** which is also used to make non-stick pans.

- **PFAS** chemicals.

- **Parabens, phthalates,** and **phenols** in cosmetics and sun creams.

We are polluted with parabens. It's even found in **amniotic fluid**, the liquid that surrounds a foetus.[61] Parabens, phthalates, and phenols mess with your **hormones.** They can make kids start **puberty earlier** than normal.[62] Parabens also make female rats **infertile.**[63]

To avoid chemicals in your products...

- **Check the label.** "All-natural" does not mean chemical free. Teflon or PFAS chemicals are "fluoro". Look for a long name such as "per-fluoro-decalin". The label might say "paraben" or a word ending in "ethyl", "butyl", "methyl", or "propyl".

- **Avoid fragrances** and perfumes. Perfume industries have the right to guard their recipes. What the word "fragrance" actually means is "nasty chemicals". Order natural perfumes online. Anyway, we give off pheromones to attract a mate, so perfume actually makes you **less attractive** to the opposite sex.

- **Scale down.** We are bombarded with advertisements. They tell us that we need a certain product to enhance our looks. The truth is that you don't need half of the stuff that you put on your face. Whatever you do buy, make sure it's natural.

- Use the EWG website to **check** how toxic your products are on a scale of 0-10. Zero means it's safe and 10 means it's toxic.

- **Make your own** beauty products. To find out how, type into a search engine "MAKE BEUATY PRODUCTS".

- **Use body oil** instead of lotion. The oil and water would naturally separate without stabilising chemicals. Check the label still; baby oil is just as toxic as a lotion.

Bottom Line

Spend your efforts fixing yourself from the inside out. - SEE COLLAGEN, SUPERFOOD AND DRINK, RED LIGHT THERAPY, EXERCISE, WEIGHT-LOSS

Access the workbook - Health Hacker 30 Day Challenge - *AVOIDING TOXINS. Start your toxin-free journey today!*

10 POINTS TO REMEMBER

1. Ageing well depends on a combination of factors.

Spain was ranked the healthiest country in the world in 2019.[1] We can learn key life lessons from them:

- Eat the Mediterranean diet
- Get sunshine on your skin
- Sleep well
- Keep active
- Don't drink too much alcohol
- Relax

2. Every little helps.

The smallest change to your lifestyle can have an impact. The more small changes you make, the healthier you will be. You can only do your best.

3. It's not about being perfect.

Sometimes I drink too much wine and sometimes I eat what I shouldn't. That's totally fine! Don't beat yourself up for falling off the bandwagon. Just jump straight back on.

4. Don't rely on the government to protect you.

Trans fats and mercury fillings are proven toxic, but are still available in the UK until 2021. Companies replace one toxic substance with another, and we wait another decade to prove the harm caused.

5. You can have too much of a good thing.

We see this time and time again. A bit of alcohol, whey protein, meat, or sunshine is good for you. It's the over-indulgence that will kill you.

6. Taste changes.

The more you experiment with new food, the more you find healthy options that you like to eat. When you taste a lot of bitter foodstuffs like green vegetables, coffee and tea, your palette adapts to them. The more you eat them, the better they taste.

You crave what you eat. I crave broccoli for example. I know that sounds weird, but I do! Likewise, refined sugar tastes terrible to me. The less of a food you eat, the less you like it.

7. We are all unique.

Diets don't work for everybody in the same way. Our gut microbiomes are all unique, so we like different foods. Pay attention to what makes you feel good.

You might feel tired after eating. That means that your body is working really hard to digest your meal, and it's draining your energy. Smelly gas is another sign that your gut is having digestion difficulties.

Think back to what you ate and write it down. Over time, you will see that a common foodstuff is triggering your symptoms.

8. Your mind and body are linked.

The gut and the brain constantly send messages between themselves. Good nutrition makes depressed people happier, as does regular exercise. That's because exercise makes your brain release pleasure hormones.

The better you look after your body, the sharper your mind, and the less chance you have of developing dementia.

9. You are the master of your own destiny.

Your health is in your hands. You have the power to avoid disease and age well. Value yourself enough to make healthy choices.

10. It's an upward spiral.

When you feel crappy, you want to eat crap food. When you feel healthy, you want to eat healthy food. The more exercise you do, the less alcohol you want to drink, and the healthier you want to eat. The better you feel, the healthier you want to be.

Change your lifestyle because you deserve to live to a HEALTHY, HAPPY 100. Make health your priority. It's your most valuable asset!

ABOUT THE AUTHOR

Curious Kirsty, Teacher & Author

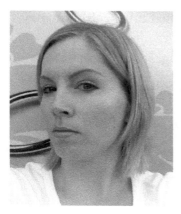

Curious Kirsty is an author and teacher from Surrey, England. She has lived in Argentina, Colombia, France and Taiwan. She speaks fluent Spanish and French.

After a lot of hard work, Curious Kirsty is finally satisfied with her body and state of mind. She gets a thrill out of motivating people to be healthy.

She has an inquisitive nature. If you ask her friends from school, she was always the girl with her hand in the air waiting to ask a question.

She loves London, and takes every opportunity to visit museums and galleries there.

To learn about Curious Kirsty's writing journey, visit…
www.curiouskirsty.com

Follow **Curious Kirsty** on Instagram, where you can watch her videos and rate her circus skills. @curiouskirsty

Can I help you?

Sometimes, we need a little push to kickstart our health journey.

If you would like private health coaching, send an email to…
info@curiouskirsty.com

Include a subject heading… PRIVATE COACHING

Can you help me?

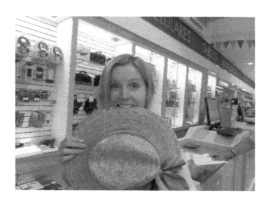

Can you think of **anyone** who would really benefit from reading this book?

Wouldn't it **feel fantastic** to be the person who helped kick-start their health journey?

Peter Diamandis said…

> **"The best way to become a billionaire is to help a billion people."**

Please help me to fulfil my dream. **Pass this book** on to a friend.

If you have enjoyed this book and want to thank me. Please **write a review** on Amazon. I would love to read how I helped you to become healthier.

Understanding how your body works makes it easier to be healthy.

In the same way, understanding how your mind works makes it easier to be healthy.

Healthy mind, healthy body.

The next instalment in your health upgrade is in the making! Keep your eyes peeled for…

MIND YOUR HEALTH

To learn more about the next instalment in the HEALTH HACKER series, visit <u>www.curiouskirsty.com</u>

If you have any questions or comments, please email me at…
info@curiouskirsty.com

Thanks for your support!

Because life tastes better when you feel fantastic every day.

Curious Kirsty

Live like you mean it!

Lightning Source UK Ltd.
Milton Keynes UK
UKHW021427020720
365920UK00002B/203